——— THE ———
SUIT BOOK

EVERYTHING YOU NEED TO KNOW
ABOUT WEARING A SUIT

CLARE SHENG

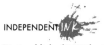

First published 2018 by Independent Ink
PO Box 1638, Carindale
Queensland 4152 Australia

Cover design by Alissa Dinallo
Internal design by Independent Ink
Typeset in 11/15 pt Adobe Garamond by Post Pre-press Group, Brisbane
Cover model Lee Carseldine
Styled by Elle Lavon
Suit and shoes by Calibre
Photography by The Portrait Store
Illustrations by Jo Yu (PQ Fashions)

 A catalogue record for this
book is available from the
NATIONAL
LIBRARY   National Library of Australia
OF AUSTRALIA

978 0 648 2865 0 9 (paperback)
978 0 648 2865 1 6 (epub)
978 0 648 2865 2 3 (kindle)

Disclaimer:
Any information in the book is purely the opinion of the author based on her personal experience and should not be taken as business or legal advice. All material is provided for educational purposes only. We recommend to always seek the advice of a qualified professional before making any decision regarding personal and business needs.

ACKNOWLEDGEMENTS

Big thanks to my mum. She started the business as a single mother, knowing very little English, and with only a couple of thousand dollars, but a lot of guts.

Over the years, she worked tirelessly for 12 hours a day, seven days a week managing and growing the business. At the same time, she put me through a private school and university. She is the pillar of my strength, my inspiration and my hero.

What initially began as a necessity, a way to put food on the table, had become a passion project for mum. She loved helping men and women feel good about themselves by making them look their best. She enjoyed tackling every garment as a project, working out ways to take it apart and putting it back together.

Throughout my school years, I helped out at the shop every school holidays, by making deliveries, buying lunch for everyone, washing the mugs and everything else to do with running a small business. I saw how tired Mum always was, and I particularly noticed how a lot of people treated her as if she was invisible.

Etched deep in my memory is an incident that happened when I was helping her during the school holidays. A high-end boutique shop saw me walking towards them with an armful of altered garments for delivery. They opened the door for a client who was in front of me, and then closed the door on my face as I was nearing them, so I had to push the door open with my body while holding their garments.

People took advantage of my mother's kindness, and they looked down at her because of her race and her profession. She never took it to heart; however, she never wanted me to take over the business, and go through the same hardships that she did.

After being disillusioned with my first career as a pharmacist, and leaving the industry, I didn't know what to do with my life. Never would I have imagined that I'd take over the business and grow to become so passionate about it. I'm glad that I am now able to promote our business, raising its social status so that clients see us as a valuable service. Most of all, I'm able to bring Mum's hard work, skills and passion into the spotlight, making her clients and peers look at us in a new light, and to showcase all of her achievements.

My team, thank you – for without you *The Fitting Room* would not function. You all work so well together – treating each other with respect and as a family, sharing knowledge and learning together. I am so proud of all you, and I consider you Australia's No.1 team! Thank you Mylene, Madeline, Sheena, Sam, Yvonne, Huong, Mary, Winnie, Yan, Julie, Lin, Han Wei, Elaine, Dianne, Fabienne, and Sofia.

Big thanks to my cousin, Jo, for creating the amazing illustrations while wrangling a baby and running a business. She is a true artist.

And thank you to my friends who have supported me and listened to me stress and complain about the book-writing journey. Your faith in me has meant so much! I'm incredibly lucky to have friends and colleagues who act like my cheer-leading squad, helping me get through all the ups and downs of entrepreneurship.

I want to also acknowledge the DENT team. Andrew Griffith is an amazing author mentor, who has guided me through each step of making this book possible, and Mike Reid for being a good friend and solid support through the last 12 months.

Lastly, I want to thank my husband, Chris. The rock behind my madness, the Yang to my Ying, you are always quietly supporting me, encouraging me and keeping me calm.

PRAISE FOR CLARE AND
THE FITTING ROOM

[Clare's] dedication to Brisbane is well recognised and I thank you for being passionate about providing jobs to local residents and contributing strongly to the city's economy.

Graham Quirk
(Lord Mayor of Brisbane)

I have been using The Fitting Room for a number of years now and have found them to be extremely experienced and highly knowledgeable with suits and how it should fit. Their staff are attentive and efficient, making it very convenient to have any of my new garments altered and old garments mended. I am confident in recommending them to any of my colleagues and clients.

Peter Chisholm
(Director, Morgans Financial Ltd)

Thank you TFR! I have been working with you for over a decade now and wouldn't dream of using anyone else! As a business owner who's been in the fashion industry for 15 years, specialising in high-end men's suiting, I know and understand the fine workmanship and service that is required when dealing with delicate fabrics and structured garments.

Elle Lavon
(The Executive Stylist)

Exceptional. The Fitting Room offers high-quality tailoring and alteration services. The work is of a very high standard, precise and cost effective. I always recommend The Fitting Room and will definitely be using their services in the future.

Alexander Gonano
(Westpac)

Clare Sheng is a phenomenal businesswoman, owner and now friend – having developed a truly fantastic business relationship with her. We rely on Clare and her business, The Fitting Room on Edward Street, so that our business, Tom James, can even function. Clare has the three qualities that ensure success as a business and as an individual: ambition, energy and integrity.

Ben Mayer
(Manager, Tom James Tailors)

In the short time I've known Clare, her team and her business, I have constantly been floored by the core dedication to customer care matched with a willingness to identify a changing industry ready for disruption and positive change. You only need to talk to Clare for a few moments to understand her passion, vision and genuine nature in delivering supreme services within an industry that has up until now not been regarding favourably or rarely spoken about. Clare's willingness to disrupt the mindset and misconceptions of the general public towards her services will undoubtedly serve The Fitting Room on Edward well into the future. This change has clearly been led by Clare – inspired by her mother's challenging journey into a business often looked down upon.

Nathan Schokker 'That Guy'
(Entrepreneur)

Clare and her team have proven themselves to be the leading authority in suit tailoring in Australia. Because we only work with high-calibre clients and sell extremely high-quality suits, I can only trust her to deliver the best advice and results, every time.

Aung Lynn
(Director, Canali and Mitchell Ogilvie Menswear)

I've had multiple garments altered, repaired and modernised at The Fitting Room, and I have ALWAYS been very happy with the workmanship, service, time and cost. I'll never use another tailor in Brisbane again, and neither should you.

Rhys Cockram
(McGrath Estate Agents)

I've dealt with these guys for a while and they always deliver for me with great customer service. Would recommend them to anyone!

Mayowa Adeniyi
(Manager, InStitchu Brisbane)

I love being able to bring in all my new purchases to The Fitting Room, whether it be casual shirts, business shirts, pants or a suit, and leave it in the hands of the professionals, because I know I will have a great finished product in the end. When I get compliments on my clothes now, I know that 'fit' is one of the main reasons. I have recommended The Fitting Room's style and clothing alterations services to many of my colleagues and friends, and many of them are now also addicted to well-fitted clothing.

Ryan Clancy
(BHP)

Don't take your garments anywhere else!

Jaime Burnell
(Asset Manager, DEXUS)

The Fitting Room is best for delivering excellent service.

Tamer Abasiry
(Manager, Hugo Boss)

Clare has worked hard with her team to establish themselves as THE DESTINATION for tailored services. Her extensive knowledge of garment construction has, on many occasions, made all the difference to clients across both gender lines, age demographics and various body profiles to create a tailored finish to rival any made-to-measure product. In my opinion, they have set the benchmark on what tailoring should look and feel like.

Beverley Sekete
(Ex-manager, Hugo Boss and Armani Collezioni)

One cannot underestimate the confidence, the power and the shift in identity that occurs when dressing in clothes that not only feel good but also look good. The Suit Book *is a comprehensive 'how to guide' which enables you to enhance your identity, move into another peer level and accelerate professional career all through the power of a suit. Not just any suit, but a suit that fits you extraordinarily well, is matched to you now and also propels you to where you are going in your career. Implementing the teachings from this book has helped me excel in business and especially at times when I needed that extra firepower. I was shocked and pleasantly surprised by how big a difference it made to my confidence, how I 'showed up' and ultimately how I am perceived.* The Suit Book *is a must read for anyone who wants to look good and feel great in their own skin and their clothes. It's for people who want the edge and have a strong desire to succeed and scale their professional career.*

Dr. David Dugan
executive business coach

CONTENTS

INTRODUCTION

'Clothes make the man.'

Mark Twain

WHY I WROTE THIS BOOK

This book has been a long time in the making. Previously known as Brisbane City Clothing Alterations, *The Fitting Room on Edward* has been helping Brisbane men look well dressed for over 19 years.

I never thought I would see myself working in the family business, as I had no ambition to do so growing up. However, after working five years as a Pharmacist, there was no job satisfaction, and I felt like I was not making enough of a difference in people's lives.

I would see my mum working her butt off every day, but she was happy, enjoying every moment. I realised her happiness came from helping to improve the way people felt about themselves. If you ask any successful man what is the secret to their energy and confidence, they will tell you 'It is wearing a well-fitting, power suit'. That was when I decided to join my mum and help her.

For the last seven years, I have worked with thousands of men, tailoring their suits, and helping them look their best. Every man should aim to have a wardrobe full of 'power suits'. A well-tailored suit is like a coat of armor, it provides the wearer with a feeling of confidence, helping them to make an impact in the world. A well-dressed man usually receives the promotion, lands the deal, and gets the upgrade.

Every time a client brings in a new suit to be altered, I get a little excited. Every person's body shape is different, and each suit is like a puzzle for me to solve, working out the delicate touches and seams we'd need to add to make the suit look amazing on the wearer.

Each time the client picks up their suit, I love watching their faces light up when they see the difference a bit of tailoring can make. They stand up straighter, they lift their head, and they feel more confident.

However, I realised there was a gap in knowledge. A good suit is an essential part of every wardrobe, yet so many men still don't know how to shop for, alter and style their suits. All the essential knowledge every suit wearing professional should know. So, I started writing regular blogs to answer these questions, as well as publishing *The Fit Guide – How to Look Good in Every Suit*, which is in its third print run. But, the questions kept coming. That was when I decided to write this book – *The Suit Book*.

In this book, I will decode the process of buying and wearing a suit, reveal why even the most expensive garments will look cheap if they're not fitted properly, and how you should care for your suit like an investment.

I hope you will enjoy reading it as much as I enjoyed writing it, and please contact me on clare@thefittingroomonedward.com if you have any questions or suggestions.

About The Fitting Room

Since taking over the family business in 2011, I have grown it into a seven-figure business, employing 20 staff. *The Fitting Room on Edward* is now the largest independent alterations tailor in Queensland, Australia. Our clients include CEOs from major banks, politicians, and influencer personalities. We have also landed partnership deals with men's retailers such as Ermenegildo Zegna, Hugo Boss, Canali and dozens more. Each year, we perfect over 20,000 suits.

In 2017, I co-founded *The Modern Gentry*, a new–age society for men and women to fine-tune skills ranging from contemporary etiquette to the art of dressing well and dinner party chat. Being a gentleman is a journey of growth that is shaped by personal experiences. Monthly social events are held with guest presenters, where the aim is for people to meet other interesting new people and discuss a variety of subjects that may challenge their way of thinking. Ultimately, we want to create a place where men and women can find answers to the everyday things Google can't help them with – like whether that paisley tie is really a good idea, or how to impress at their next work presentation.

The events canvas a range of ideas and experiences because a well-rounded gentleman is like a well-fitted suit – it's the small details that matter. Those who become members are more likely to have new doors opened for them, both personally and professionally.

In 2017, I was honoured to be the winner of the Nick Xynias Multicultural Young Business Person of the Year, and the Small Business Champion Awards in Fashion. I also received a special mention in the Lord Mayor's Business Awards in Business Innovation.

PROLOGUE

You only get seven seconds to make a first impression – so are you making it count?

You may think it's shallow, that you shouldn't judge a book by its cover, but it doesn't change the fact that everyone gets judged on their appearances. Humans are visual beings – it's just how our brains are wired. When you meet someone for the first time, they will most likely look you up and down and form an opinion of you based on the way you are dressed. Seven seconds is your first opportunity to show others that you are someone worth listening to.

A good suit will make you look like you are at the 'top of your game', and it makes a powerful statement about what you can achieve.

When you get up and get dressed each morning, do you emulate someone confident like 'Harvey Specter' from the TV series, *Suits*? Or do you feel drab and uninspired like 'George Costanza'. Even if you are not genetically blessed like Chris Hemsworth, you should wear clothing that will uncover the best version of yourself, instead of hiding in an ill-fitting sack.

How you look paints a story of who you are. Do you want to be the guy who looks like he just rolled out of bed and grabbed the first thing he could reach in the dark, often an ill-fitting, poorly made outfit that hasn't been ironed? Or do you want to look like someone who is put-together, confident, a powerful go-getter who puts attention into his grooming and clothing because he is someone who is driven and who will do whatever it takes to be the best in all he does.

How you dress says a lot about you. If you take pride in your appearance, it shows your attention to detail, your respect for the person you are meeting, and confidence in your own skin.

The clothes on your back are like your suit of armour. They make you look good and feel invincible. A good power suit will help boost your confidence and intimidate your opposition. Being well groomed and well dressed also shows self-respect and respect for others. It shows that you are serious about your clients, your job, and your life in general. Your appearance is a reflection of your company, your work and what you represent.

HOW THIS BOOK CAN HELP

Many men hate shopping for suits because:

* They don't know what type of suit to buy;
* They have no idea which style is suitable for their shape;
* They don't know what the differences are between suit brands and styles;
* A good suit costs thousands of dollars, and sometimes even $10,000, but why?
* They often feel pressured by the sales people and end up buying things they never liked in the first place.

Once they have the suit, there are even more things to consider:

* Finding a good tailor to help them look their best in their suits;
* Which is the right suit to wear for different dress codes and occasions?
* How can I look awesome and yet still feel comfortable in the suit?
* How do you look after and maintain the suit?
* How often should you get it dry cleaned?
* What do you do once the suit has been damaged or dirtied?

Unless you have a live-in butler or a personal stylist on call, these things can be overwhelming and confusing.

This is where this book will provide you with all the information you need.

I have identified four key areas of the suit-wearing process, to help you buy better, wear better and maximise the wear of your suits. By following these simple steps, you will soon find that your whole wardrobe will be filled with quality, well-tailored clothing that you will look forward to putting on every day, and the best thing is that you'll feel awesome wearing them.

The four key areas discussed in this book are:

Section One: Dress according to your style, purpose & body shape

Firstly, look in the mirror and understand what is body shape and identify your uniquenesses, in order to work out what styles suit you. You'd be surprised at how doing this will allow you to streamline your wardrobe, and how much time you will save when next buying a new suit. In this section, I will show you what to look for, which styles to choose and when to wear them.

Section Two: Find the right suit for every occasion

Why have ten cheap suits that don't fit, and then feel horrible every time you put one on? Instead of chasing 'fast fashion' – the contemporary term for certain styles that are manufactured quickly at low prices to follow a certain trend at that time – and buying 'seasonal colours' that don't look good on you, you should buy better. Build up a collection of good-quality suits and have them tailored to fit. Feel the confidence and power it gives you each time you put one on. The golden rule is always 'quality over quantity'.

In this section, I'll tell you how to acquire perfectly fitting suits in good-quality fabric that won't break the bank.

Section Three: Have your suit altered with confidence

The most important part of any suit is the fit. It doesn't matter if the suit costs $300 or $3000 – if it doesn't fit, it will look unflattering and ultimately make you feel uncomfortable and less confident. In this section, I will break down how jackets, trousers and shirts should fit every person (of every shape), how to get it fitted, and how to find the right tailor for the job.

Section Four: How to care for your suit so they last longer

Make the most of your suits by cleaning and caring for them like they are your best friends, because they are important investments. It is crucial to maintain your suit after each wear and to get it cleaned properly. In this section, I'll discuss the many aspects of maintenance to maximise the life of your suit.

In section five, I'll talk about the 'return on investment' of owning and wearing power suits, as well as how to behave like a modern gentleman once you have the look down pat.

So let's get started …

⌘

WHY A 'POWER SUIT'?

In the last ten years, the emergence of modern tech firms, such as Google, has given rise to a new breed of casually dressed, modern professionals. Icons like Mark Zuckerberg and Steve Jobs never wore a suit, as they found fashion a distraction, opting to wear a uniform of plain t-shirts every day.

However, if you are not yet a multi-millionaire or eccentric CEO, can you afford to dress in a shabby fashion in the work place?

And think about this, why do doctors wear a white coat? Or why do pilots wear a pilot's uniform, or why do lawyers always wear a formal dark suit in court? As soon as they put on their 'uniforms', it makes them do a better job. These 'uniforms' help put them in an elevated frame of mind to achieve more. And by wearing an appropriate style, this also ensures that others trust them in their roles.

Frank Abignail, the famous con man who inspired the movie, *Catch Me if You Can*, knew that how you looked was the key to how people reacted to you. When he was wearing a pilot's uniform, he *was* a pilot. When he put on the outfit, it gave him the confidence and the illusion of success, power and capability, which made everyone else trust him, even though he was just a teenager at the time.

This is what a 'power suit' should do for you.

Apart from the obvious reason, such as you only get one chance to make a first impression; there are many more reasons to wear a power suit to succeed in the work place.

Below are five examples to showcase how wearing a power suit everyday will change your life.

Command leadership

Don't ask for attention and respect, command it. Obama wore only handmade bespoke suits custom designed for him. Nothing prepares you for getting ahead in your life like wearing your power suit. In most cases, the best-dressed person in a room of strangers instantly becomes the voice of authority and power. If a man in a bespoke tailored three-piece suit walks into a room with confidence, people will automatically think, 'this guy knows what he is doing'. They will subconsciously look to him for leadership.

Exude confidence

Fake it or make it. Who is more likely to get an upgrade on a flight, take a Ferrari out for a test drive, or get a better hotel room – someone dressed in a blue t-shirt and jeans, or someone dressed like Don Draper? A power suit reduces your self-doubt and gives you the confidence you need to close that deal. Imagine back to when you were little – did you have a favourite outfit? Maybe it was a Superman costume, or a pirate's outfit. How did it make you feel when you put it on? Did it make you feel like you *were* Superman, and that you could achieve anything you wanted? That's how a power suit should feel when you have it on – you are ready to overcome any obstacle.

Be in control

You understand the power of appearance, and so you always make sure your suit is impeccably styled and pressed, which then translates into your actions. Your handshakes become stronger and more confident. Your voice is firm and louder. You know what you like, and you don't settle for second best. People will remember you, even after meeting you only once, and they will pay more attention to what you have to say. You will be memorable, and people will think, 'this guy's got his act together'.

Have a winner's attitude

The formidable character 'Harvey Spector' says in the show *Suits*: 'That's the difference between you and me. You want to lose small; I want to win big'. A powerful suit is a reflection of your attitude to strive to be a winner, and it puts you in the right frame of mind to ensure that you accomplish this. Don't have dreams, have goals.

Be media ready

Be prepared for any situation life may throw at you, such as an impromptu presentation, an unscheduled photo op, meeting someone new, or bumping into your ex. You will look your best in every scenario. A well-cut suit will also make you look in better shape than you are. When the boss needs to bring a client in for an important meeting, he will pick you over someone else who is not properly dressed.

But if you need more reasons as to why dressing better will improve your life, here they are.

* You only get one chance to make a first impression.
* Dressing well shows maturity of the wearer.
* The clothes you wear and the way you groom yourself changes the way other people hear what you have to say.
* When you're wearing quality well-fitting clothes, it gives you a reason to stay fit to be able to keep wearing them.

- Your tailor will remember you and alter your clothes to fit your style without prompting.
- Men will stop to admire your look on the street.
- Women will stop to admire your look on the street.
- Your boss will take more notice of what you have to say.
- You are more likely to get upgrades at hotels.
- Your chances of getting the job or promotion are increased.
- Clients will find you more trustworthy to take care of their business, because you take pride in your appearance.
- Dressing well shows self-respect.
- Strangers will give you the benefit of the doubt.
- A well-fitting suit makes you look like you are in great shape, even if you are not.
- You will look confident and fabulous when you run into an ex.
- Your handshakes become stronger and more confident.
- You will be more likely to get an upgrade on a flight.
- You will start to seek out formal events to wear your beautifully tailored suits.
- You will become better at accepting compliments.
- You will be more likely to be able to take that Ferrari out for a test drive at the showroom.
- You'll always look good in photos.
- You'll never have to worry about having nothing to wear again, because everything in your wardrobe is well curated.
- You will inspire others to dress better.
- People will pay more attention to you when you are making a presentation.
- You will look forward to colder days so you can wear your coats, hats and gloves.
- You will begin to understand the power of appearance.
- Your peers will respect and listen to you more.

- When you go shopping for clothes, *you* can dictate what you want to buy, not the assistant.
- People will remember you more, even after meeting you only once.
- You will become familiar with different types of fabrics on suits.
- You will understand what pleats, vents and braces are.
- You will reconsider the hem and sleeves length on all the garments you already own.
- You will start investing in pocket squares, cufflinks and other accessories that will change the look of your outfit.
- Friends and colleagues will start asking you for style advice.
- You won't have to worry about not finding something that fits off the rack, because your tailor is your best friend.

⌘

SECTION ONE

DRESSING ACCORDING TO YOUR STYLE, PURPOSE, AND BODY SHAPE

'Looking good isn't self-importance; it's self-respect.'
Charles Hix

COMMON MISTAKES MEN MAKE

Australia is a young country, and as such, not many people understand the true history, value and potential of a good suit. The amount of readily available information on how to wear and fit a suit is few and far in between. Here are some of the most common mistakes men make when wearing a suit.

Wearing an off-the-rack suit and not having it tailored

The less experienced may buy a suit straight off the rack and wear it as it is. I've heard many excuses from such buyers – they think a suit off the rack is how a suit is supposed to look, and they shouldn't mess with the style.

This is a big mistake.

Mass production and the concept of 'one size for all' came into existence during the First World War, when the uniform production had to be sped up to keep up with demand. Before that, when you needed new clothes, you'd go to a dressmaker to have it made, which meant that every garment was perfectly fitted every time.

Off-the-rack suits are *meant* to be altered to fit each individual person and their shape and size. If anyone tries to tell you otherwise, I would stop taking any fashion advice from them.

Buying the wrong size

I know quite a few large-sized men who like their suits to be loose fitting. They buy their clothes a little bigger than they need, thinking they can hide their insecurities in the extra fabric. In fact, this has the opposite effect on big guys. Big suits make them look bigger than they actually are.

Thin guys also often buy a bigger suit, thinking it will make them look filled out, when in fact they look like they are propping up a tent. There are also the guys who buy suits slightly too small, trying to look fashionable, thinking that this is the way suits are supposed to fit. However, suits in a catalogue or on Instagram are styled according to the look the fashion company wants, and are usually too small for the men wearing them, or they have been pinched in by pegs to look smaller. In reality, these suits would probably split as soon as the men lifted their arms or tried to sit down.

Wearing perfectly tailored suits should make you look like you are in better shape than you actually are.

Too long or too short

Too often I see pants bunched up at the hem, or jeans turned up a few times, because men don't know that their pants can be shortened. There are also those who wear their trousers shorter, because the shorter length is in fashion right now. However, without tapering the width of the trouser legs to balance out the proportions, they look like schoolboys who have outgrown their trousers.

Similarly, when the sleeves on the jacket are too long, they can make the wearer look especially short, ruining the look of a perfectly good suit. If the sleeves are too short, they look equally badly dressed.

Ill-fitting business shirt

Many guys do not put enough thought into the business shirt, so when they take off the jacket, the look falls apart straight away. Too often, the shirt is too big, too long, too wide and not properly ironed. The sleeves get rolled up because they're too long, or to appear as if you are 'getting into business'. When in fact, rolling up your sleeves in the office actually steps down the formality of a look straight away, making you look stressed out and overly casual. It's best to keep this look for the weekends, when wearing a casual shirt paired with casual pants.

The business shirt is an essential part of your outfit and needs to be perfectly tailored for the same reason as your suit. The sleeve length should be just right, so you don't need to roll them up. The torso of the shirt should be well fitting for a clean and tidy appearance. If it's too tight, the buttons will pull at the front. If too loose, the shirt will look like a parachute.

I'm going to lose weight

There have been many times when I have heard the excuse: 'I don't want to alter it now, as I'm about to lose some weight'. In answer to that, I suggest they focus on how they look and feel in that moment.

Do you want to feel good in a well-fitting suit, or do you want to feel miserable and useless for not having lost this weight yet? Forget about always losing another two kilograms – embrace your body now. Ill-fitting clothing makes you look in worse shape than you actually are. As mentioned above, a well-tailored suit will make you look like you are in better shape than you are. Imagine the difference you will feel when you are not wearing a suit that is a bit too tight or too loose.

Wrong suit for the wrong occasion

Understanding dress codes is a very important element of dressing well. It can be embarrassing when you show up to an occasion wearing the wrong outfit. Only recently, I saw a guy catching a bus after work who was wearing chinos with a velvet tux jacket. It may be a stunning-looking jacket, but a tux jacket is best left for black tie events, not for everyday work.

And if you choose to turn up for a business meeting in jeans and a t-shirt – thinking that you are a young entrepreneur and don't need to dress up – if the clients don't know you, they will think that are you are being disrespectful and are inexperienced. Is this the first impression you want to make?

Making sure you wear the correct attire will help you feel more comfortable in your surroundings, look more cultured, and give you more confidence.

Wearing worn-out clothing

Hole in the trousers; buttons missing; rip under the arm – you might think that people won't notice, but they *do* notice. You should either get it mended or throw it away. Don't wear it as it is and hope no one else will notice. Good personal grooming speaks volumes to your professionalism, self-respect and general personal hygiene.

Chasing 'fast fashion'

No explanation needed. 'Fad clothing' or 'fast fashion' is expensive, wasteful, and it only lasts one to two seasons. Buying quality clothing that are classic and timeless will pay for itself over time. Fashion trends come and go, but a tailored fit never goes out of style, especially when wearing quality clothing that has been made with care. It feels good knowing that you are wearing your favourite suit, which fits like a glove, and it makes you look and feel amazing. No doubt, you'll receive compliments every time you wear it.

Too many accessories

It's best to keep your accessories to two or less. It's hard to pull off multiple accessories without looking like a magician or a hustler.

Coco Chanel famously said, 'Before you leave the house, look in the mirror and take one thing off'.

Understated elegance speaks volumes compared to wearing too many accessories, which may come off as gaudy. Classic items such as a vintage watch and silk tie will complement every outfit.

⌘

WHAT IS YOUR WORK STYLE

The power suit can mean something different for everyone. While one may like to wear a dark three-piece fully bespoke suit, another may like a double-breasted suit in a bright colour, or even a nice sports jacket with tailored trousers.

What your personality and line of work is, will determine what your power suit looks like. Build your style profile around your work life, social life and personality. Take into account the area that you spend the most time in. For most people, it's work. So let's focus on some appropriate suits to wear in various settings.

Work examples:

> I am working in a conservative and traditional setting: e.g. law firms, investment firms, government, where the people I deal with are also conservative and generally older than me.

These working environments are where you are expected to put on a full formal professional business suit every day. You are trying to climb the corporate ladder and want to dress for the job you want. Dark colours and block colours are preferable. Your suits need to be perfectly tailored and maintained to show your professionalism, and to reflect your competence and self-respect. Make sure your suit fits well without being too tight or too short. Remember that you are more likely to be working with older people who are more traditional, and who may still prefer the professional way of dressing. Imagine showing up to an important board meeting wearing an oversized suit you are drowning in, the board members will no doubt immediately think of you as a rookie and put less trust in anything you have to say, whereas a suit that is loud, tight and short may also give a negative impression.

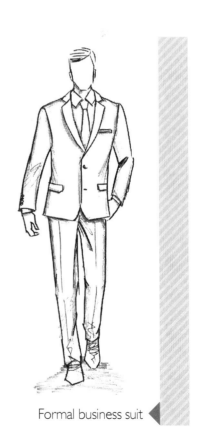

Formal business suit

> I am working in a dynamic field: e.g. sales, marketing, working with a variety of people who embrace creativity, energy and personal flare.

You may still need or like to wear a suit each day, but you have the option to dress it up or down, and you can be more creative with it. You can buy suits in different colours such as light blue, light grey, or even purple. Try out different styles – one button, double-breasted, or unconstructed suits. Paired with different accessories, such as bright ties and pocket squares, it will demonstrate that you have put thought into your appearance and it shows your creativity. Suits can be altered to look more fashionably fitted, e.g. the torsos can be made a little tighter, the legs slimmer and trouser hems shorter. You may even like to mix and match different looks, such as wearing a sports coat with different coloured trousers, tied in with a good mixture of accessories. However, make sure you still have a good pair of shoes that are well maintained, closed in and polished. The most important point is that even though the garment is more casual, the look only works if everything is immaculately tailored and maintained.

> I am working in a young and vibrant field: e.g. start-up companies, tech firms, where there is no strict dress code. I still want to dress to impress and make myself feel good.

There are many young firms that are taking up the trend of a smart casual workplace. People like Mark Zuckerberg and Steve Jobs have been leading the way in casual dressing at the workplace.

However, unless you are a famous billionaire, I think it is still important to dress well to make a good impression. How you dress at the workplace affects the way people see you. Wearing a dirty t-shirt and jeans with holes is not good social etiquette, and your peers or your clients will be less likely take you seriously. In smart casual firms, it's a good idea to wear very smart clothes, such as well-tailored jeans (no holes) and well-fitting dress shirts (tucked in), completed with a leather belt and sports coat.

And as with the other examples, dress for the job you want. When client/investor walks in, they'd more likely defer to the person who looks most like he is in charge – for example, the guy in a tailored sports coat verses the one in t-shirt and cargos.

Of course there are more than just three categories of work-places, and you may like to take elements of each look to create something of your own to best suit the one you work in.

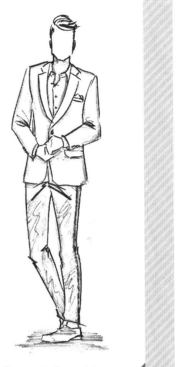

Sports jacket with jeans

⌘

WHAT IS YOUR BODY SHAPE

Men can have many different body shapes. Recognising what shape you are is the first step to helping you buy better suits that will *complement* your body shape. Some of the most common shapes are rectangular, inverted triangle, round, and triangular. Let's look at each more closely.

Rectangular

If you are a rectangular shape, it means that your shoulders are quite even with the width of your hips. This is a very common body shape for men, and if you're lucky enough to be a rectangular shape, you are most likely to be able to fit into a suit bought straight off the rack – with the exception of perhaps needing to have the length of the sleeves and trouser hems adjusted. Rectangular-shaped men can wear most suit styles, including single and double-breasted suits. You may like to have your jackets tapered a bit through the centre of your waist, to create a more stylised shape.

Inverted triangles

The next most common shape is the inverted triangle. This means that you have wide shoulders and a small waist, where the base of

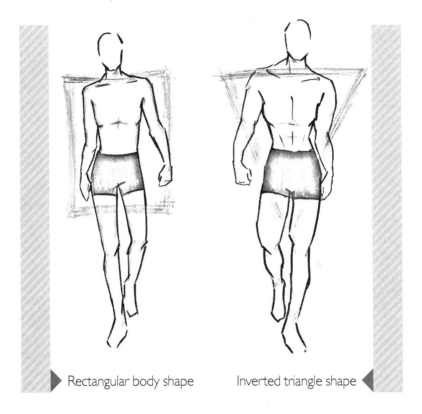

Rectangular body shape   Inverted triangle shape

the triangle is the shoulders and the tip is at the hips. This shape is common on guys who go to the gym often and who like to work on their upper section. It's recommended they find a suit that will balance out the waist and remove emphasis from their wide shoulders. The point of a suit is to create balance in the overall shape. If they wear their clothes really tight, they will look out of balance and top heavy.

So if you have an inverted triangle figure, try to wear your suit loosely tailored in the waist area, instead of skintight. Unstructured jackets with less shoulder padding are also good for this shape. Stay away from wide lapels and big patterns, which will emphasise your wide shoulders. You will most likely require alterations on off-the-rack suits, or have it custom-made.

Round

Then we have the round body shape, where the midsection of the body is more prominent compared to the shoulders. When buying suits, opt for sizes that fit the waist and tummy first, then have the rest adjusted to fit. Try to go for simple lines and dark solid colours to create a more slimming look. Your jacket should float on top of the body, not be skintight or too loose – both of which can make you look bigger than you are. A dark coloured suit with a bright tie or pocket square is ideal. Round shaped men sometimes have trouble finding trousers to fit nicely around the waist, therefore braces or suspenders will be helpful in keeping the trousers on the waist throughout the day.

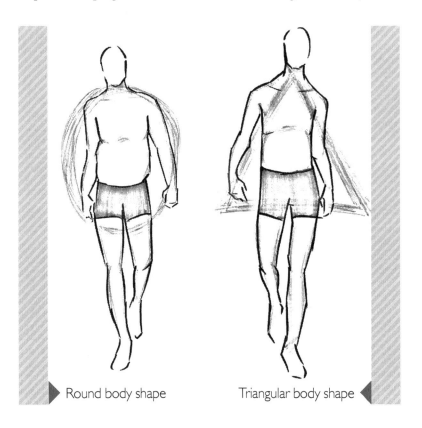

Round body shape   Triangular body shape

Triangular

Finally, there is the triangular body shaped men, with narrow or sloped shoulders and thicker set waist and hips. The tip of the triangle is at the shoulders, and the base of the triangle is at the hips. You may want to try and broaden your shoulders by finding structured jackets and take attention away from your midsection. Try to avoid unstructured clothing that does not give you definition in the shoulders, instead go for wide lapels and thick shoulder pads.

⌘

WHY ARE COLOURS IMPORTANT

Have you ever worn an expensive outfit that fit perfectly, but somehow it just didn't feel right? That's probably because you were wearing the wrong colour for your skin tone. Choosing the correct colour and shade can make a world of difference to your appearance.

However, it is not just your skin colour that you have to consider. You must also take into account your hair colour, brow colour and 'warmth' of your skin tone.

There are at least 12 palettes of colours suitable for different skin tones. The colours are separated into 'warm' and 'cool'. In the warm range, they are then separated into 'spring' and 'autumn' colours. Then in the cool range, they are separated into 'summer' and 'winter'. Within the seasons, there are at least three more grades of shading.

Some examples are:

Warm colours

- yellow
- orange
- red
- yellow-orange
- red-orange
- red-violet

Cool colours

- violet
- blue-violet
- blue
- blue-green
- green
- yellow-green

Each person has one to two palettes they can wear, which suit their complexion and make them look amazing. Choosing the right one is tricky. So spend some time testing out your colours to find what makes you feel more 'you'.

Most people buy suits in grey and blue, which are safe colours to wear. However, did you know that there are many different shades of blue, such as navy, royal, light blue? These varieties can look good on some complexions and not so great on others eg. people who are very fair should avoid pastel in the majority of cases. If you are having trouble, it's worthwhile contacting a personal stylist to help you out.

Here are two examples of how colours can make a dramatic difference to your look, and knowing what works and what doesn't is key in highlighting or dulling your features.

I once heard a story about a lady who worked in a very conservative corporate office. She and everyone around her always wore black and grey – they dealt with multimillion-dollar clients – and their clients always wore dark colours too. However, one day she was very hungover after a big night, and so she wore what she actually liked to wear, which was a brightly coloured outfit she would otherwise never have worn to work. Throughout the day, everyone complimented her on how fabulous she looked. Even though she felt miserable from the hangover, she actually looked brilliant.

Another example is about a client of mine who loves suits, and who is very particular about the way he dresses. He has pale skin, light golden hair and golden eyebrows. He always used to wear perfectly fitted suits, but in colours that made his skin look dull, such as grey and green. When he was styled at one of our *Modern Gentry* events, he was given a light-cream pair of trousers, a white shirt and a blue blazer. This combination of colours instantly brightened his face, and it brought out the colour in his cheeks. A gold pocket square helped to tie in with his golden hair, and it completed the look. The transformation was instant and astonishing.

It just goes to show that wearing the right colours can do wonders for your 'look'.

⌘

UNDERSTANDING YOUR
UNIQUENESSES

If you are extra tall or shorter than most, you may have difficulty finding the right length off the rack. Be prepared to put aside some money to have all your purchases altered to fit. The most important things to look for in any of your purchases and alterations are the proportions and keeping everything in balance. Here are some tips when shopping for the right fit.

Tall guys

If you are tall, try and find a suit retailer who make a 'long cut'. These cuts are designed for people who are tall and thin, without an increase in the actual suit size. I have had clients who bought their suits a couple of sizes bigger, just so they could get the right length in the sleeves and pants. However, to make the suit then fit the client's frame, we had to reconstruct the whole suit. The suit was then the right size, but the button position and lapel length were not in the right proportions and the whole suit looked out of balance.

It's best to look for a suit that is your size, and then have the lengths adjusted. *Tip:* New trousers can usually be lengthened by up to 5cm, and jacket sleeves usually by 3cm. Unfortunately, if the jacket length is too short, it can't be made longer.

The telltale sign of an ill-fitting jacket is when the buttons on the jacket sit too high on the body. Instead of buttoning at the waist, the jacket buttons at the chest, and therefore the whole upper body will look out of proportion, almost like the man is shrugging his shoulders all the time. The first button on a two-button jacket, or the second button on a three-button jacket should sit level with the smallest part of your waist.

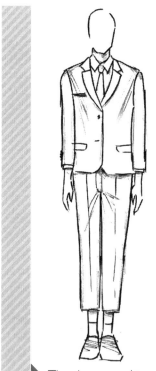
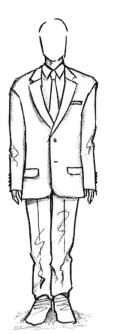

The sleeves and trouser on this suit are too short, and the jacket sits too high on the body.

The suit is too long for this guy, the lapel is too low, and sleeves and trousers are too long.

Short guys

Similarly, I have seen men avoid buying suits in the correct size, thinking the sleeves and pants are too long. They then buy a size that is too small because the length seems to fit better. The sleeves and the hems on the trousers can easily be shortened, and the jacket length can be usually shortened by up to 2.5cm. However, if the suit is too small, the amount that can be let out is very limited. We often recommend customers return their suit and purchase the correct size.

Once shortened, make sure you have the legs or sleeves tapered, so the whole look remains in proportion. Check that the same button rule applies as for tall guys – where the first button should sit level with the smallest part of the waist. To check the length of the jacket hem is the correct length, relax your arms by your side. The hem should line up with the knuckle of your hand. We will talk more about fit in Section Three.

Know your uniquenesses

You probably don't realise that the majority of the population have different lengths between their left and right arms and/or legs. There are also many different shoulder shapes – sloped, very slighted, or square. Many people also have their shoulders at different slopes, which could be due to being right or left-handed, having an injury doing repeated exercises, or occurring naturally from birth. Different leg lengths could be due to hip injuries, and different arm lengths due to shoulder injuries.

It is very important to know and recognise if you have different arm or leg lengths, and to tell your tailor before you have alterations done so that the clothes are altered to look balanced when worn. To wear a suit well, you should know everything about your body.

With jackets, it can simply be a matter of shortening one sleeve a little less than the other, so both arms look the same once altered.

We had a client who always wore his suits a little big, so he had never noticed that his shoulders were sloped differently. That was until he bought his first Hugo Boss suit to wear to his wedding, which needed to be professionally altered. The client had square shoulders, so we did a nip in at the neck, which revealed the fact that his left shoulder was slightly higher than his right shoulder. This in turn made the sleeve lengths look ½ centimetre different on each arm. It took a while to explain to him that it was not the suit that was uneven, but it was his shoulders.

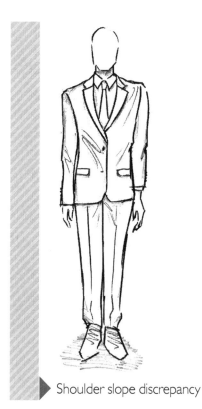

Shoulder slope discrepancy

After we took a photo of him from behind and showed it to him he realised the difference. To solve the slight imbalance, we removed half of the shoulder pads on the left-hand side, so both sides look balanced. We *could* also have added a half layer of shoulder pad on the right to lift it; however, the client's shoulders were already square, so it was best not to accentuate them even more.

Shoulders

Most manufactured suits are cut with slightly sloped shoulders. This is the equivalent of the standard slope of the majority of the population. However, there are also many men that have squarish shoulders, where the slope is not very prominent, or men that have very sloped shoulders where the shoulders drop steeply from the neck to the top of the arm.

The guys with squarish shoulders will often notice a bubble form at the back of the neck, this is common, and can be easily rectified with alterations.

Men with very sloped shoulders will often find extra fabric gathered under the arms of the jacket. One solution is to opt for extra shoulder padding, which helps to widen their shoulders, and it gives them a very confident and powerful look.

There are many other examples of uniquenesses. Most times, we can make you look balanced and well tailored with alterations. There are some cases where custom made suits is a better option.

Legs

When it comes to buying trousers, it is also very important to understand your own shape. Are you quite muscular with a prominent behind and thick legs? Are you quite slim with a small behind and skinny legs? If you have a more prominent behind and muscular legs, common problems are your trouser pockets are often flared out, or the pants sit a bit low on the waist and your behind can show when you bend down. You may also find that your trousers get worn out more quickly in the seat and thighs.

For guys with a large behind, it is a good idea to buy high-waisted trousers with a long crutch length, also known as the rise, as this will fit you better and reduce the 'plumber's crack' situation when you bend down. Buy trousers in a size that fit the hips and thighs instead of buying trousers according to your waist size, and then have the waist taken in to fit. If the seat on the trousers is too tight there is very little scope to adjust the fit.

It's unlikely that you will be able to wear the very tight/slim leg trend if you have muscular calves, as it will make your legs look out of proportion. If you try to taper the legs too much, the fabric will hug on your calves. Not only is this uncomfortable, it is also very difficult to walk in, and the fabric will be riding up to your knees all the time. A high-waisted classic fit, perhaps with a small pleat at the front and cut to the right length is ideal for muscular men.

For men with slim legs, make sure the legs of your trousers are a slim fit, but not too tight. You want to look balanced instead of emphasising your skinny legs.

One very important rule when buying clothes is to always fit to the largest part of your body first, as the rest can be tapered, and we will talk about this again in Section Three.

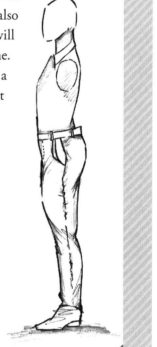

Large bottom and thighs

In conclusion, know that 99% of men do not look like a store mannequin, so prepare a budget of $100–$200 on clothing alterations to finish the look of your suit. Wearing clothes bought straight off the rack is not a good option if it doesn't fit properly.

It is also a good idea to tell your tailor about your uniquenesses if any, especially if they're subtle, as your tailor might not be able to pick them up at your first meeting. So make sure you highlight what's different about your figure, as this also ensures that you don't end up spending more money on further alterations later down the track. Your tailor can then make a note of these uniquenesses on your file – and remember that everyone has 'quirks', so you should embrace them.

⌘

DECODING THE DRESS CODES

How you dress says a lot about you. It speaks to your personality, sophistication, and your sense of style. It is therefore very important to dress well and dress appropriately for different situations and events. When you are not wearing the right outfit for the specific event you are attending, it can be quite embarrassing.

We have previously touched on the appropriate attire to wear to various workplace scenarios, and so here I will give you a few more guidelines on how to pick the right outfit for other occasions – workplace attire suggestions are also included.

Formal business

Dressing for a formal workplace or work function is not that hard, and you can easily pull it off with a good suit. A formal workplace or a work function requires the attendants to carry themselves in a dignified manner, and since time immemorial a well-fitting suit has been the epitome of formal functions. The suit should be in bold dark colours such as black, blue or navy. Fit is very important in this case, and your suit should be cut to fit you perfectly. It shouldn't be too tight or too short, like the fashion at the moment, nor should it be over-sized.

The suit should be paired with a dress shirt in lighter colours, such as white or blue, for a clean-cut look. French cuffs on the shirt give a sophisticated yet modern look. You should wear a dark-coloured necktie for the complete formal look. Finish the look with brown or black leather shoes, and a belt in the same colour. The jacket usually has a notch lapel and two flap pockets. The trousers should have belt loops or adjuster tabs.

Smart business

Many workplaces are beginning to embrace informal wear at the workplace and at work functions. This is when you can pull off your most fashionable looks by wearing shorter trousers and firm-fitting

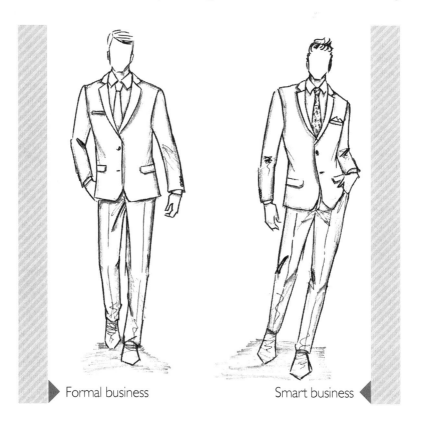

Formal business   Smart business

suits. You can also now wear your chinos and coloured shirts to the workplace. Pair these with a sports coat or a blazer for a simple yet sophisticated look. As always, even your casual clothes should be well fitted and tailored to perfection.

Since you are at the workplace or at a work function, closed leather shoes or loafers are preferred. Open-toed shoes and sandals are not welcomed at the office space, or at specific work functions, and as such, they do not make up the smart business attire. And t-shirts, loud Hawaiian shirts, or clothes with cartoon characters are best left out of the office and any functions – unless of course it is themed as such – as they undermine the wearer and the workplace.

It's also a good idea to keep a tie and suit jacket at work for any emergency client meetings where you'd like to dress to impress.

Lounge suit

This dress code is common for business events taking place during the day and in the evening. It can also be worn for social functions with some degree of formality such as wedding receptions and lunches. For these events, you can opt for a dark suit worn over a French-cuffed white shirt with no tie.

Cocktail attire

Cocktail attires became prominent at the beginning of the 20th century, when the wealthier and more fashionable members of the society started wearing them to social events. Cocktail attires are semi-formal in nature and allow their wearer to be free to enjoy the event. When picking an attire for a cocktail party, it's always advisable to check with the host on how 'casual' the event is going to be, before you show up in your distressed denim.

Cocktail events also provide you with an opportunity to dress up and stand out. A great way to dress for a cocktail event is to go with a tailored suit, a white dress shirt, a stand-out tie, and dress shoes such as Oxfords. You can accessorise the outfit with a pocket square and fresh boutonnieres. For less formal events, you can go with jeans and a blazer. The jeans, however, should not have tears.

Smart casual

The objective with this clothing style is to combine formal and informal wear into one impressive package. So if you think your jogging bottoms paired with a blazer qualify for smart casual, then you're definitely wrong. You can wear your chinos with a long-sleeved shirt and closed-toed shoes. You can also wear your jeans

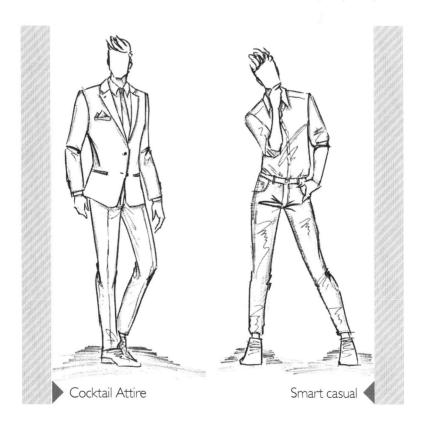

Cocktail Attire   Smart casual

with a well-tailored button-down shirt. The jeans should be dark and without tears for a smart look. T-shirts under a blazer are also acceptable, as long as they're smart-looking and in good condition.

Black tie/formal

Of all the dress codes available, dressing for a black tie is the most rigid. Black tie attires have been worn since the 1800s, when the upper-class British men started easing away from the stuffy attires that were worn by members of the British high society. Black tie attire is very strict, and for this you can only wear a tuxedo or dinner suit, in a shawl or peak lapel. The lapel should be faced with satin or gros-grain. It should be worn with a satin bow tie that is also black.

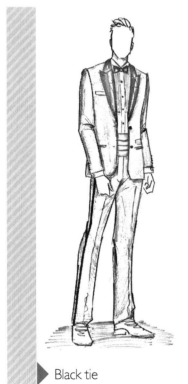

The shirt for this dress code should be a dress shirt with stud closures and a wing collar. You should also wear a black low-cut waistcoat or cummerbund to complete the look. The trousers you wear to a black tie event should be in the same colour as the jacket, which is usually black. A satin strip on the outside seam of the leg is essential. Black and to some extent velvet are the traditional colours of a black tie event, and you'd be wise to stick to this colour code.

The more daring may wear a dark navy suit with black satin lapel, or even a velvet suit. A white suit with black lapel is NOT a good look, and

Black tie

it will make you look as if you are going to a high school formal. Finish the look with black socks and black, formal leather shoes.

Not knowing what to wear for different occasions can be difficult, and choosing the wrong outfit can be embarrassing. The tips and tricks throughout this guide will help you avoid any embarrassing fashion faux pas, ensuring you feel relaxed and confident at every occasion.

⌘

HOW TO BUILD A WINNING WARDROBE

Having a well-curated wardrobe makes getting dressed in the morning a breeze. When you invest time and money in shopping, choosing, tailoring and maintaining your suits, anything you pull out of your wardrobe will make you look good, for any occasion.

Imagine your dream closet, where every garment is hung up in a well-organised way, and all pieces match each other, with different sections for your work, casual life and special occasions. You'll be able to get dressed for whatever event presents itself to you – no stress or confusion. Wouldn't that be an easier way to begin each day?

Here are seven quick tips to building a winning wardrobe.

Buy well

Quality clothes in a fine fabric will last longer, be more comfortable to wear, and look better. Choose one to two mid to high-end brands that suit your shape and look, and invest in building a professional wardrobe to last the test of time. Build up your wardrobe over time, acquiring at least one quality suit per year. It won't be long before you have a wardrobe full of beautiful garments.

Get it altered to fit

It doesn't matter how much your clothes cost, if they're not tailored to your body, they will look cheap and unkempt. Invest a bit of time and money when your suit needs clothing alterations. A well-experienced tailor like *The Fitting Room* will help you elevate your look by making sure every line is tailored to complement your shape, while providing comfort.

Maintenance

Clothes that are worn directly on the body should be washed or dry-cleaned every three to four wears, and jackets every three to six months. This prevents discolouration and makes the clothes last longer. Any ripped seams and holes should be mended immediately by a professional alterations service, to avoid looking careless and unobservant. We will talk in depth about maintenance in Section Four.

Don't follow trends

Trends should not apply to a professional wardrobe, because 'fast fashion' usually means cheap, disposable clothing that fades, rips, and even loses its shape easily. Don't waste time buying something you can only wear for 6–12 months, then have to go and purchase another piece when it starts to look worn or goes out of style. Wearing classically tailored and styled clothing also shows maturity.

Stick to the same colour scheme

Having too many different colour palettes in your wardrobe means you will end up spending more time each morning trying to match outfits. Instead, choose two to three of your favourite staple suit colours, e.g. navy, light grey, and black, and build a collection of complementary coloured shirts and ties to match. Don't forget to only buy clothing and accessories that suit your skin tone, instead of buying different colours to suit your moods.

Accessorise

This is when buying well and to a colour scheme is important again. Choose timeless pieces to complement your staple looks. For example: a good-quality leather workbag, three to four professional belts, leather shoes in brown and black, simple jewellery, watches and lapel pins – these can all elevate your look. Keep the total number of accessories to one to two pieces worn at one time. Silk neckties are also a good investment – buy them in classic colours such as maroon, navy and grey. A pocket square finishes the look but should never be in the exact same colour as the tie.

Build a signature look

There is nothing more time saving than building a signature look, because everything in your wardrobe will already match. Family lawyers may like to wear more colours and softer lines, whereas corporate lawyers could wear sharply tailored suits in lighter shades. If you shop for your personality or area of work, anything you pull out of your wardrobe will match and look good.

Now you know the importance of buying a suit that fits, and how to build a functional wardrobe. In the next few chapters, I'll discuss how to look for and purchase pieces to add to your professional wardrobe effectively, and how to make every suit your 'power suit'.

⌘

SECTION TWO

FIND THE RIGHT SUIT
FOR EVERY OCCASION

*A man should look as if he had bought his clothes
with intelligence, put them on with care,
and then forgotten all about them.'*
Sir Hardy Amies

THE DIFFERENT TYPES OF SUITS

Once you have recognised your suit style, have studied your shape and know your colours, you have your 'occasions' sorted and are ready to build your wardrobe, it's time to find your power suits.

In this section, I will elaborate on the differences between the plethora of suit styles, different suit suppliers, and to help you choose the most appropriate suit for you. I will also give a detailed description of the many and varied additional suit components, and I'll discuss the important stages of wearing a suit, why you need to build a style and purpose profile, as well as buying the correct size for you.

Basic suit

This is usually a two-piece or three-piece suit in a pure wool or wool blend. Most often, these suits have a notched lapel, which is occasionally peaked. They can come in single or double-breasted, and with flap pockets. There is sometimes a narrow ticket pocket as well on the right-hand side above the flap pocket. The trousers are plain with a flat front or pleated front, and most often they will have belt loops on the waistband. The hem is finished plain or with a cuff.

It is a good idea to get two pairs of trousers when you buy a work suit, as the trousers always wear out faster than the jacket.

The colours should be navy, and charcoal, with some patterns such as pinstripe or check. Wear these with shirts in any (matching) colour such as white, grey, and blue. Try and avoid a black suit, as it makes a very bold statement and is usually reserved for funerals or evening time.

Dinner suit

The dinner suit is also known as a tuxedo. A proper tuxedo always comes in navy or black (not white). The lapel is faced with satin or grosgrain, in a shawl or peak shape (never notched). The pockets are jetted (no flap, or have the flaps tucked in) and there is no ticket

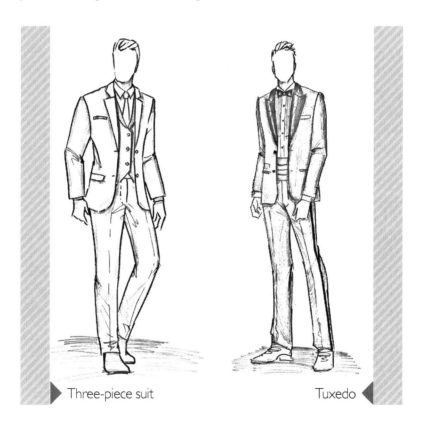

Three-piece suit   Tuxedo

pocket. The buttons are covered in the same fabric as the lapel – they should not be plastic, horn and especially not metal. The trousers always have a satin strip running down the side of the leg, and are often cuffed.

Always wear your tux with a dress shirt, which has a pleated or textured front, with studs or a covered panel to hide the buttons. Wear your trousers with a cummerbund in the same colour as the lapel, to cover the waistband, or use braces to hold up the trousers. Never wear a belt. Finish the suit with a black or white self-tie bow tie. Your shoes should be polished dress shoes, not monk straps, which is too casual.

Tails

You wear tails when the occasion calls for a morning suit or white tie. The jacket has a long, rounded back like a tail. All other elements are similar to black tie, except that the bow tie or wide neck tie must always be in white, hence the 'white tie'. The trousers are grey and pleated, and the look is finished with a top hat. You will often see a white waistcoat worn with the suit, and the trousers are often cuffed. This is an extremely formal look, and you will rarely see 'tails' worn in Brisbane.

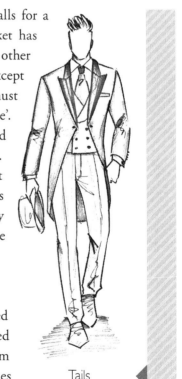

Tails

Sports jacket

The sports jacket is usually half lined for more breathability, and constructed with a softer fabric, usually from cotton, linen, wool, and sometimes blends. There is less shoulder padding for a more relaxed look, but it can be tailored to fit you more stylishly. It comes in many different colours, especially bright colours such as red and light blue. Details, such as elbow patches and different types of pockets (patch or flap), can be added and played around with. Usually there are no matching trousers with sports jackets, so you can wear them with jeans and chinos for a dressed-down look, or wear them with suit trousers to slightly tone down the look for after work occasions. A pocket square is a nice finishing touch.

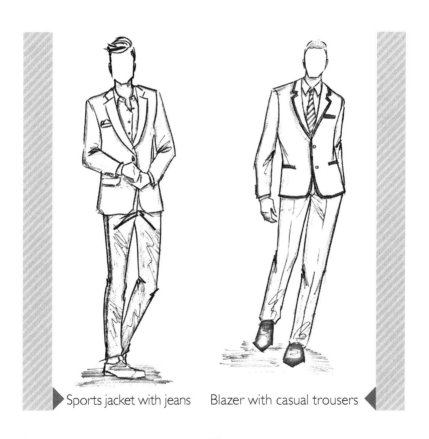

Sports jacket with jeans   Blazer with casual trousers

Blazer

Blazers are a descendent of naval uniforms and should be in dark blue. When you imagine a blazer, think 'school uniforms'. The shape is generally squarish with wide shoulder pads, notched lapel, and the pockets are patched on. It is usually made with dense and heavy wool such as worsted wool serge. Gold metal buttons, gold stripes and epaulets are common features of a blazer. Blazers go well with check trousers or light-coloured chinos. Overall, the look is 'preppy', and can be worn as an upscale sports jacket.

⌘

ALL THE EXTRA BITS ON A SUIT

When buying for a standard suit, there are many components to consider, and the specifics that make up a suit's overall structure should also be given some thought. Here are some details about these additional aspects of perfecting your suit styling.

Jackets

Single-breasted

This is the most casual style. The one-button jacket only has one button at the front, and the button sits lower than the first button of a two-button jacket. It is usually positioned in the lower part of the smallest part of the waist. This jacket is most suitable for slim guys and for a casual occasion.

The two-button closure jacket is the most common and suits the majority of body shapes. The first button sits around the smallest part of the waist, with the second button around the tummy. The second button should never be done up.

The three-button jacket is not in fashion right now. It has a shorter lapel and the buttons sit much higher. This style is suitable for guys with a flat tummy, but it will accentuate a large girth. The first and second buttons can be done up, but never the third.

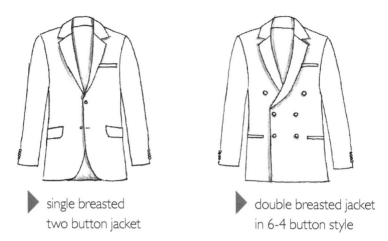

▶ single breasted
two button jacket

▶ double breasted jacket
in 6-4 button style

Double-breasted

Thanks to the 'Kingsman' movies, double-breasted jackets are coming back into fashion with a vengeance. When worn well, it will make a bold statement. 'The DB', as most people like to call it, is a more formal look, with the buttons done up at all times. To avoid looking old-fashioned and boxy, it should be worn fully tailored, and worn with confidence. There are a few different styles of DBs, which consist of different types of button configurations.

The first number is the total number of visible buttons on the outside, and the second number is the number of buttons that are done up. The top two buttons are usually set apart.

Above is an example of 6–4 style.

Three-piece

The three-piece jacket includes a waistcoat that is made in the same fabric. This jacket is more traditional and looks elegant and old-fashioned. However, this style definitely screams 'power'. The last button on the waistcoat should be left undone.

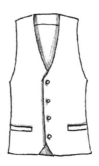

▶ Waistcoat for Three-piece

Lapels

Notched – The most common lapel, appropriate on business suits, blazers and sports coats. It can also be in different widths.

Peak – This is usually found on wide-width lapels, ranging from slim to wide, and seen on double-breasted and dinner suits. Some fashion suits also have the wide-peak lapel as a feature.

Shawl – This is found exclusively on dinner suits, and sometimes on fancy smoking jackets.

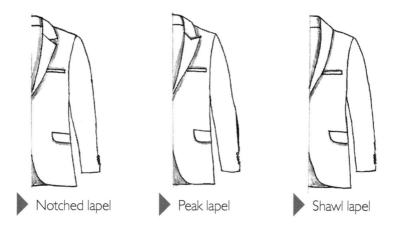

▶ Notched lapel   ▶ Peak lapel   ▶ Shawl lapel

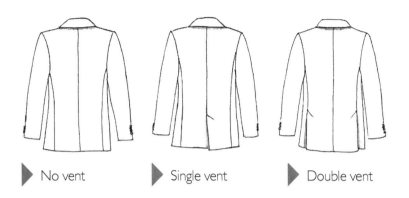

No vent   Single vent   Double vent

Vents

No vent – This is usually seen on tuxedos/dinner suits.

Single vent – The most casual look, it is traditionally designed for horse riding. It is not suitable for guys with a large behind.

Double vent – This is the most common style, vents should sit flat against the body. If it's popping out, the jacket is too tight.

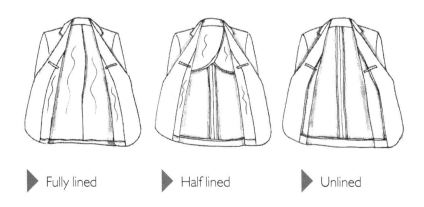

Fully lined   Half lined   Unlined

Lining

Lined – Most suits are fully lined on the inside. Natural linings, such as silk and cotton, will be more breathable than synthetic polyester lining.

Half lined – The back section of the jacket is not lined, as seen on sports coats in very soft fabrics. This style drapes better on the body, has a soft look and is more breathable in summer.

Unlined – Only seen on the most casual of jackets, made in cotton or denim fabrics.

Pockets

Jetted/besom – Only trimming on the pockets can be seen, as there are no flaps, or the flaps are tucked in. It is a more formal look, reserved for dinners suits.

Flap – It is the most common pocket style, seen on most suits. The flaps can be tucked in for a jetted look.

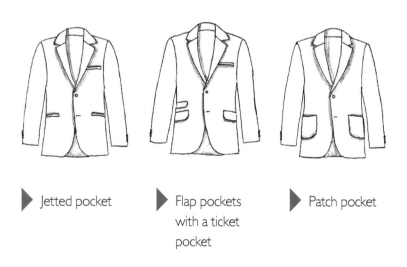

▶ Jetted pocket

▶ Flap pockets with a ticket pocket

▶ Patch pocket

Ticket pocket – It is a small pocket on the right front of the pocket, above the flap pocket. It got its name from when English gentlemen wanted an extra pocket for easy access to their train tickets.

Patch – This is when the pocket is patched on top of the jacket, and the whole pocket is visible on the outside. Very casual look reserved only for blazers and sports jackets.

Trousers

Flat front

Most trousers either have a flat front or a pleat front. Flat front is the most common. As the name suggests, the fabric is completely flat in the front. It gives a tapered look and is suitable for men of slim or standard shapes.

Pleat front

Pleat trousers often have one to two folded pleats in the front of the trousers. These give the wearer more room in the seat and thighs, and therefore this style of trousers is suitable for guys with larger behinds and thighs. It's also a sophisticated and traditional look.

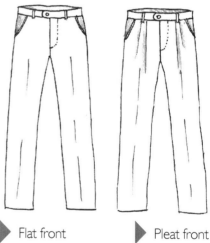

▶ Flat front   ▶ Pleat front

Waist features

Belt loop – Most trousers come with belt loops. As adding a belt tones down the formality of an outfit, remember to never wear a belt with a tux.

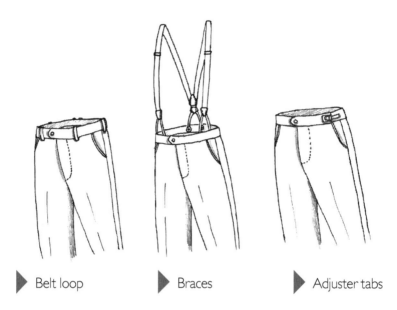

▶ Belt loop   ▶ Braces   ▶ Adjuster tabs

Braces – Never wear braces as well as a belt. However, you can leave the buttons and belt loops on the same pair of trousers, so you can choose which one to use. Usually there are six buttons on the inside of the waistband, where braces or suspenders are attached to hold the pants. This is perfect for guys without a defined waistline, to help hold the trousers in place.

Adjuster tabs – Extremely popular right now, tabs are made with the same fabric as the trousers, paired with buckles on each side of the waist. They can be pulled to tighten the trousers up to 3cm, this is handy so you can release it when sitting down and need more room, and then you can tightened them up when you are standing.

⌘

NOT ALL SUIT FABRICS
ARE MADE EQUAL

A suit's fabric is one of the most important components that affects the price of a suit. Ranging from fully synthetic, which is much cheaper, to wool, cashmere and silk blends, which may cost hundreds of dollars per metre. When you are wearing a suit made from synthetics, it can be quite obvious and can be spotted from a mile away. The fabric is very stiff, usually shiny, and does not hug the body. Wool is generally advisable for everyday wear, as it is more breathable and sits better on the body. Finer wools graded 'Super 120s' and above will drape even better, and they elevate the overall look of the suit and add sophistication. These finer wool blends are delicate fabrics that are not for everyday wear, but they make the wearer look a million bucks.

Synthetics

Polyester, Rayon, Acetate

These are all man-made fabrics and are generally cheaper to produce and to buy. The weave of the fabric is usually very tight, making it not breathable on the skin. The fabric is also less soft to the touch; sometimes it even feels scratchy when you rub your fingers on it.

Because of the stiffness of the fabric, suits made with a synthetic fabric are usually made with the 'fused' method, which means that the suit doesn't curve well against the body, ultimately giving a very rigid look. Overall, a synthetic fabric is far inferior to a natural fibre. The only advantage is that this fabric is harder wearing, especially in the crotch area, meaning that it will last longer. It is also less likely to wrinkle due to its stiff nature.

Wool

Wool is the most common natural fibre used in suiting. It can be woven to form many different types of fabrics. When the wool is in the 'super' category, e.g. Super 100s, 120s, up to 180s, they are referring to the number of times the wool is twisted when it is made. The higher the number, the finer the cloth and more expensive it is.

Super 160s and 180s may feel amazing, feeling like liquid silk against your skin; however, they are less durable than a standard fabric. Suits made with these fabrics are not meant to be worn on a day-to-day basis. If you are lucky enough to buy a suit in 160s plus, try to wear it no more than once per week, and leave it hanging on a good coathanger to air out before storing. This gives the fibres a chance to set and go back to their natural shape.

Cotton and linen

Cotton and linen are also derived from natural fibres, and they are popular in casual suiting. The fabric is more breathable and suitable for wearing in the warmer months in Australia. However, these suits wrinkle easily, fade more readily, and are not stretchy in nature. Therefore, they may change shape over time. They also don't curve around the body as well as a wool suit. When buying cotton and linen, make sure you only stick to casual and loose-fitting styles such as sports jackets.

Lining

Suit linings are usually made with polyester and acetate. These are again synthetics and not breathable. Higher quality suits may use silk as their lining, which is a far superior fabric therefore this will reflect in the overall cost of the suit. Have a look at the label on the inside pocket to find out what materials your suit is made out of.

Determining the fabric choice of your suit will come down to budget, occassion and to a degree, climate. I would recommend choosing the best possible fabric and with the right care your suit will be an investment.

⌘

FUSED SUITS VS. CANVASSED SUITS

When people talk about a suit being 'fused' or 'canvassed', they are referring to the way the jacket is made. The front of the jacket is always supported by a piece of stiffening fabric, made with horse hair (canvas) or fusible (fusing). The reason that support is used in the front only, is to give the wearer a very flat and structured look, hiding bumps and filling out hollows. The back of the jacket and the trousers are always draped fabric with no added structural support. Lining is always used on suit jackets, unless it's a casual summer sports jacket. Trousers are often lined down to the knee, to increase the life of the trousers, and it helps the fabric to drape better.

Fused

To make suiting more affordable for everyone, fusible suits were invented. Instead of hand-stitching the canvas to give a suit shape, a synthetic layer is glued (fused) to the inner side of the suit fabric, giving it structure. However, with any stiff fabric, it doesn't mould well to the body.

Fused suits works well enough for most people who have flat chests. On guys with large pectoral muscles or a protruding tummy, the fused jacket will not curve around the body nicely and will never

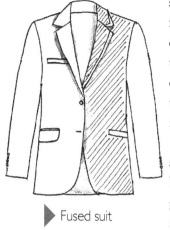

Fused suit

sit well. Another downside to the fused jacket is that the glue can break down over time. Overheating from the drycleaners or inferior glue can cause the fabric to bubble away from the fusing. This cannot be fixed and means the suit will need to be replaced.

However, that doesn't mean you should not buy a fused suit. Most brands make them in a decent quality, good enough to wear for work, or to make a fashion statement.

Canvas

Before fusible suits came along, all suits were canvassed by hand. The canvas is the piece of fabric made from horsehair that is hand-woven loosely onto the fabric of the jacket in the front panels and the collar.

The canvassed suit is the most labour-intensive to produce. It requires high craftsmanship, hundreds of man-hours and is therefore the most expensive option. The fabric of the suit almost floats on top of the canvas and therefore drapes more softly.

In this manner, the suit fabric drapes better and has a softer look, while the canvas helps to hold the shape of the front panel. The canvas will mould to the shape of your body over time, which means it will look better with each wear.

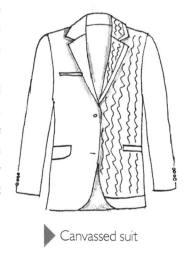

Canvassed suit

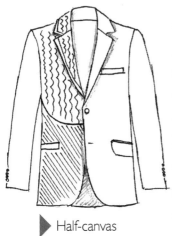

▶ Half-canvas

Half-canvas

The half-canvas suit is a happy middle ground and is slightly more affordable. The floating canvas is stitched to the upper part of the front panel of the jacket only, to give a natural finish on the chest, while the bottom half of the jacket is fused. This helps to keep the price down, and yet it still provides a better and more contoured look than the fused jackets.

The key thing to look for when buying half-canvased suits is the craftsmanship. A cheaper manufacturer may cut the canvas differently to the fabric, and this could cause bubbling in the fabric. And check that the hems and seams are all finished properly, with straight lines and sharp corners. The suit will not look good if it is made carelessly.

⌘

WHERE TO BUY YOUR SUIT

Buying a new suit can be a confusing and overwhelming affair. There are so many options, but which is best for you? Should you buy off the rack, or custom-made? One must also take into consideration the timeline and budget for alterations.

If you have a rectangular shape, then congratulations, you'll most likely be able to pick a suit off the rack with minimal alterations. The rest of you will need to budget for alterations when buying your suits. If you know you have a couple of uniquenesses, as explained in Section One, such as being extra tall, then you may need to invest in custom-made suits.

Below I list the five most common ways you can buy a new suit and what the differences are.

Off-the-rack

Most people prefer to buy off-the-rack suits. You can try on different shapes and cuts, touch the fabric for quality, and you are able to wear the suit right away. There is a huge variety of options for buying off-the-rack suits, ranging from $300 wool blends to $6000 Italian-made cashmere. The reason for the variation in cost is mostly due to the quality of the fabric, the manufacturing country, as well as the craftsmanship of the tailor putting the suit together. How a $300 suit is made, could be incredibly different to how a $6000 suit is made, and you will feel the difference when you are wearing it. If you are not a conventional shape, or if you want the suit to be heavily tailored, then be prepared to put away around $100 to $250 for alterations.

Every brand varies in their style, cutting and costs. Brands targeted at younger, fashion-conscious men will stock smaller sizes and slimmer styles, whereas more traditional brands will carry styles that are roomier and suitable for round-shaped bodies. Within each brand, there will also be different cuts, such as classic, slim and super slim, varying in long and short styles.

I'd suggest you try on as many types and brands as you can initially, and find a style and brand that suits you the best and that you feel confident and comfortable in. Once you have found the magic brand that fits you the best, buy the suit in several colours, and try and purchase your suits from the same brand again in the future, because you know their suit styles are suitable for you. Afterwards, make sure you visit your tailor to get them to check the suit and make sure it is fully tailored to your shape.

Most people would need the jacket sleeves and trouser hems adjusted. Inverted triangle and square shapes would usually need the torso tapered. Round-shaped men may like the trousers tapered and the shoulders squared.

Online tailor

There are many online tailors emerging on the men's fashion scene. These businesses offer less expensive suits, as they're usually based overseas. Do your homework and make sure the tailor is experienced, they know what they are doing, and find out exactly what the fabrics are like. If you are after a matching set of groomsmen suits, or just want something different for a party, online ordering may be the way to go.

Make sure you get a comprehensive list of required measurements from the business, and have a local tailor measure you professionally. It is a good idea to send them pictures of yourself from different angles to ensure that they cut the suit to your body shape.

However, beware – you get what you pay for. Most of these suits are made with an inferior fabric and are likely to be fully-fused. The styles are cut off a standard block. If you are an unconventional shape, don't expect a perfect fit straight away. Unless the tailor making the suit is performing personal measurements, it will be highly unlikely that you will get a good fit. If the suit doesn't fit, you will also have to fork out extra alteration costs.

Made-to-measure and custom-made

There are now more than a dozen custom-made tailors in Brisbane, and many more all over Australia. These 'tailors' are essentially well-trained sales people who will help you choose a style, fabric and construction that suits you, and then have it made by their suppliers overseas. The suits are usually made within four to six weeks and sent to the store. If there are any additional adjustments required, they will send it to a local tailor to be altered.

Prices can vary from $500 per suit to $5000 plus per suit. The price is determined by the craftsmanship, country of origin, brand, construction and quality of fabric. For example, a $500 suit will likely be fully-fused or half-fused in a standard fabric. Whereas a $5000 suit will be handmade, using superior wool and fully canvassed. The lower-cost suits are great for making fashion statements, for weddings, parties and to wear as work suits. Whereas the higher-end suits in luxurious fabrics make a great treat when you receive the promotion and want to look the part.

If you have trouble finding suits off the rack to suit your shape, custom-made will ensure that all your suits fit you perfectly. Just make sure you choose a brand that is well known and has good reviews from their clients. Try and obtain some samples to touch and feel the fabric, so you know what kind of product you are paying for.

The sales person is also very important, so make sure they're experienced in measuring and understand how a suit needs to be adjusted to enhance your individual shape. They should be able to help you in all aspects of creating your power suit.

Travelling tailors

In the late 1990s and early 2000s, travelling tailors were all the rage. The exclusivity of being invited by someone in the know – usually a well-dressed friend or colleague – to a five-star hotel room where you were measured and fitted by an experienced tailor, was the 'thing' to do. Travelling tailors still frequent Brisbane, and it can be quite an interesting experience.

These exclusive tailors often hail from Hong Kong or Singapore, where the suits are made. The experience is highly personalised and special. Usually the price is pretty good too, delivering suits from $400 to $800 each, and the turnaround time is generally two to four weeks.

Again, this is good value, but very similar to the custom-made suits now based in Australia. When a suit comes back from the travelling tailors and it's not right, you have to go through quite an ordeal to have it altered, returned or remade. Whereas if you go to someone local, there is a faster turnaround time and you actually get to see them regularly and can build a relationship with them.

Bespoke

Unfortunately, it is rare to come across true bespoke tailors in Australia, especially Brisbane. Bespoke suiting is an art, a skill that usually gets passed down via generations and apprentices. It is still prevalent in places like Saville Row in London, and many cities in Italy. However, in the younger countries, such as Australia, you will be hard-pressed to find a true bespoke tailor.

With the popularising of industrial production lines, cheap suits, fast fashion, and low overseas production costs, no one is taking the time to learn this traditional skill, or even to be able to find anyone to learn from. Younger men might not even know what a bespoke suit is, let alone have touched one, worn one or know of its origins.

A true bespoke suit is where a tailor takes and uses 50 plus measurements and makes a suit from scratch, using all the measurements. The suit is usually made entirely by hand (no sewing machines). The suit is fully canvassed by hand, even the buttonholes are hand sewn. You will go through more than three fittings during the construction of the suit, so each seam is perfectly tailored to fit your individual body shape. If you are ever lucky enough to have a true bespoke suit made for you, go for it. It is a worthwhile investment, and the suit can be passed down for generations if well looked after.

⌘

THE FIVE STAGES OF SUITING

Not everyone can afford bespoke suits to wear every day, and that's okay. Therefore, here is a good breakdown of the suits you *should* have in your wardrobe – these will evolve over time just as your lifestyle evolves and flourishes too.

Starter suits

You've just started your first real job and you are excited about the future, so you want to look good without spending a fortune. You want two to three suits that are sturdy, practical and not too flashy. Buy suits made from fabrics that are wool or blended wool, and avoid tacky polyester suits. Wool-blended suits with synthetics often mean that they are longer wearing, and you may even be able to throw the trousers in the washing machine. However, if you want your suits to last more than a year, it's best to have your suits dry-cleaned instead.

The downside of a synthetic mix includes the fact that it will not be very breathable, and it will usually be fully-fused, meaning it is hot to wear and won't sit as well on the body.

Choose from a range of cuts that are available, in order to find one that suits your shape the best, and get it altered to a professional fit and length – not too tight and not too loose. You want to look modern, clean-cut and well groomed, without trying too hard. This is not the time to try and look 'fashion forward'.

Your employer wants to see you as someone who respects their job enough to put effort into looking presentable. Buy suits in dark colours in shades such as navy and charcoal, with small patterns in the fabric. The muted professional attire shows your humility and willingness to work hard to get ahead. To spruce up your look for a more creative industry, or for after-work drinks, accessorise with bright pocket squares, boutonnieres and/or cufflinks.

Your haircut should be tidy and professional, and facial hair groomed.

Spend: $200–$400 per suit plus tailoring.

Promotion suits

You've got your promotion and you are going places. Now is the time to start putting more effort into your attire. Looking clean, sharp and extremely well tailored will empower you to meet and mingle with colleagues and attend those ever-important meetings. Keep a wardrobe containing all the essentials for putting together work outfits every day without the hassle of preplanning.

Make sure you have three basic suits in charcoal, blue and a muted pinstripe. Made-to-measure will ensure that your suits fit you well, and they will allow you to add your personality and flare.

Made-to-measure service is now very accessible in Australia, with more suppliers available to choose from. You can select from a large range of styles and fabrics, and you can choose your own suit style. Make sure you meet the stylist and ask them to measure you personally so that they understand your body shape. To save wasted money, avoid trying out new online tailors where you have to measure yourself, as they cannot see you to understand your shape properly – they'll make some educated guesses from the measurements given – and disasters can often happen from miscommunication or a measurement entered incorrectly.

Another way to add some personal touch is through embroidery. People often embroider the cuff of business shirts, or inside the lining of the suit jackets. You can even embroider pocket squares. This is not to show people your name, but the extra detail in your outfit makes you feel special, knowing that this suit is personalised just for you. Doing this will no doubt boost your confidence. An occasional flash of the jacket lining showing the embroidery also demonstrates to people that your suit is custom-made.

Spend: $500–$1000 per suit plus tailoring.

Manager suits

You are the manager of the office, and so you need to step up your game and look more professional. Ill-fitting, worn-out clothing is not an option. You are the leader and everyone looks up to you for guidance. How you dress reflects on the image of the office. The quality and fit of your suits are key to making a strong impression when meeting clients or showing leadership.

You no longer need to travel to Thailand or wait for a travelling tailor to get a custom-made suit at a lower price. Invest in five to ten quality suits in classic colours that are versatile, along with different shirts and ties in a range of colours from a custom-made tailor locally. Custom-made tailors take more measurements and are (most of time) better than made-to-measure tailors.

Try different shades of black, navy and check patterns. Most suits in this price range will be half-canvassed or fully canvassed, but finished by machine. The fabrics are finer, meaning you should not wear the same suit more than twice a week.

Now is also the time to invest in some well-fitting shirts. In many Australian cities, such as Brisbane, the weather is not suitable for wearing a suit all day, so you still want to look professional and well groomed when you take your jacket off.

You should have 10–15 good-quality business shirts, tailored to your shape, which will become invaluable assets in your working life. Don't forget well-matching (but not the same colour) neckties and pocket squares to create an extremely polished look.

Spend: $1500 per suit plus tailoring.

CEO suits

You are the CEO of the company – now it's time to splurge and go custom-handmade in the best fabrics available. You have no time to spend at the shops looking around for a suit, so let the expert tailors come to your office for fittings when it suits your schedule. You'll become familiar with terms such as canvassing, pick stitch and basting. You want suits that say, 'Don't mess with me, I mean business'.

With custom-handmade, every line is expertly and meticulously tailored, and you can choose from a large array of quality fabrics in the most unexpected colours and combinations. Start your collection by having three custom-handmade suits in standout colours such as dark purple, wine, or blue checks. Don't forget to also collect a variety of styles such as large lapels, shawl-collared tux, and skinny notch lapels. Having a perfectly fitted waistcoat also adds sophistication and gives you more options to mix and match your style.

Spend: $5000 plus per suit.

Bespoke suits

You've made it! You no longer need to work for money and you don't need to dress to impress anyone else. Now is the time to enjoy the fruits of your labour. When money is no object, every garment you wear is top of the range, made by the most expert hands and in the world's finest fabrics.

Bespoke suits are usually 90 to 100 per cent made by hand over three to six months and finished on a floating canvas. The patterns are not cut off a block, but they are unique and cut just for you and your measurements. This means that the fabrics are softer, and they sit perfectly on your body, even when you are moving.

A custom bespoke tailor usually receives years of training by an experienced tailor, in all aspects of the craft. They will take dozens of body measurements and note your body shape, peculiarities and preferences. The finished product will be of an extremely high standard. The attention to the details is unsurpassed – even each buttonhole is hand-sewn and each suit is truly unique. I have seen instances where clients have had one of a kind fabric woven specifically for their suit. Imagine the extravagance, but also the feeling of power when wearing a suit like that.

Spend: $15,000 plus per suit.

⌘

HOW TO BUY THE RIGHT SIZE FOR YOU

Now that you are aware of the particular 'suit stage' you are at, and have decided where you would like to purchase your suit, it's time to focus on getting the right size. And the golden rule is, as previously mentioned, to always fit the widest part of your body first.

Jacket

The most important detail to look for when you're buying a new jacket is the fit of the shoulders. The width of the jacket should sit on your shoulders perfectly, as this is the area most visible on the jacket, as well as the most difficult to alter. The edge of the shoulder seam should sit in line with the widest part of your arm. If you can see the outline of your shoulders through the sleeves, then the jacket is too small. If the shoulder pad is peeking out and there is a dent between the edge of the shoulder pad and your arm, then the jacket is too big.

Every other part of the jacket can be easily altered by a professional, such as the sleeve length, the size of the torso, the bubble in the back of the neck, as well as shortening the jacket.

The next thing to look out for when you buy a jacket is the girth. If you have a large tummy that is wider than your shoulders, then you may choose a jacket that firstly fits your tummy. This comes back to

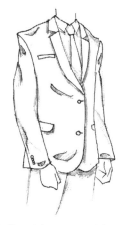

▶ Shoulders too wide

fitting the widest part of your body first. For most people it's the shoulders; however, for some it may be the chest or the tummy. If the lapel is pulling apart at the front, and your jacket is pulled open, that means the body of the jacket is much too small. Go another size up to make sure you can button the jacket up comfortably (just the first button), ensure that the lapel is not being pulled open, and that there are no straining wrinkles in the front. Then you can have your shoulders adjusted to fit.

Pants

The same concept applies for fitting the trousers. You want to fit the widest part first, whether it be the waist or your hips. If you have a small rear, then buy trousers that fit in the waist, and then have the seat taken in to fit the buttocks area. However, if you have a prominent behind, then you may want to go up a size to fit the buttocks area first. The waist can then be taken in to fit. If you choose pants according to your waist measurement, but the seat is too tight, it can't usually be let out because there is not enough fabric left in the seams.

Also, if you have a large behind, try to go for slightly higher waisted trousers. Low-waist trousers will not reach your natural waist, and they will sit too low. You'll probably feel like pulling your trousers up all the time, and your 'plumber's crack' might show when you bend down.

Again, the same goes for your thighs. If you have very muscular thighs, buy a pair of trousers that fit around the thighs first. This will still let you sit down and bend down comfortably without the risk of pulling the trousers apart. When the thighs and the seat fit well, the waist can be easily altered to fit. Usually the waistband can be taken in or let out by up to five centimetres.

Another thing to look out for when buying any kind of trousers is the shape of the seat. The length of the crutch can only be shortened or lengthened slightly, but the shape often cannot be recut. Therefore, it is imperative to check that the seat of the trousers you're trying on curves nicely under your buttocks. If it wrinkles around the middle of the thighs, it could mean that the seat is too short. If it looks like you're wearing a nappy and the crutch hangs halfway down your knees, then the crutch is much too long. Again, the crutch can only be altered slightly, so try and buy a pair of trousers that are cut to suit the shape of your derrière.

Shirt

Similar concepts apply to purchasing a shirt, as you want to fit the widest part of your body first, whether it be the shoulders, the chest, or the tummy. You want to make sure the seams of the shoulders sit just inside of your shoulders, and that there is no pulling from under the armpits.

If you have a slim torso, try to buy shirts that are slim cut with darts in the back. If you have a wide girth, try to look for shirts with a pleat in the back, which could be a centre pleat or a box pleat. These

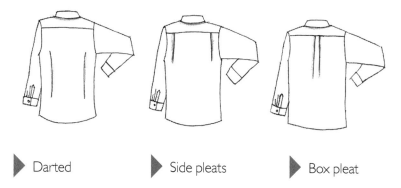

▶ Darted   ▶ Side pleats   ▶ Box pleat

pleats give you more room in the midsection area and are perfect for guys with a slight tummy. Slim guys, make sure you don't buy shirts with the pleat as it will balloon out at the tummy area.

Sleeve length can be shortened easily, but it can't be made longer. If you have disproportionally long arms, it is often quite difficult to find a shirt that fits. You can either have it custom-made, try and find a brand that makes a long cut, or go a size up and have the body altered. The last option is not ideal, as a major resize may be required.

The length of the dress shirt should not matter too much as it should be tucked in. If the shirt is curved around the edges at the hem, that means it is designed and meant to be tucked in. However, if you are wearing your shirt untucked, such as a casual shirt, you may like to have the hem shortened and reduce the curvature of the hem.

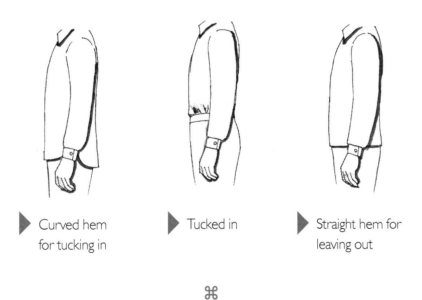

▶ Curved hem   ▶ Tucked in   ▶ Straight hem for
for tucking in   leaving out

⌘

SHOES AND ACCESSORIES

Now that you have bought your wardrobe essentials and everything looks well matched, it's time to talk accessories. You can elevate your look and make an outfit look more expensive by having quality accessories that are well matched for each look. Again, follow this golden rule: quality over quantity. Keep it simple, when it comes to ties, pocket squares and other additional decorations – wear no more than two at a time.

Shoes – Dress shoes should be worn with suits. Oxfords or brogues shoes are very suitable to wear in Australia. Boots can be worn, but they are not meant for formal occasions. Loafer shoes are best kept for casual or smart casual suits.

Belts – Only wear leather belts with suits. Keep the buckle classic and ensure there are no large, over the top logos. The colour of the belt should always match the colour of the shoes.

Ties – Unless you are going to a high school formal, please don't wear satin one-toned ties. Choose ties with classic patterns that are made in wool, cotton, and silk only. Stay away from polyester or clip-on ties.

Pocket squares – These can make a huge difference to an outfit. They should be made of silk or cotton, not polyester. Make sure your pocket square doesn't match the tie exactly, but let it slightly complement the tie colour. There are many ways to fold the square. If you want to look serious, or you are going to serious/formal event, then do a normal square fold.

Pins – Lapel pins are usually for 'secret club' members, sporting clubs etc., but they are now popular as decorations. Pins can be classy as long as there is no more than one pin on your lapel. Fake floral pins were once a trend but this is now out of date.

⌘

SECTION THREE

HAVE YOUR SUIT ALTERED WITH CONFIDENCE

'The difference between style and fashion is quality.'
Giorgio Armani

HOW TO FIND A GOOD TAILOR

I cannot emphasise enough that the fit of the suit is the most important aspect of an outfit. It doesn't matter if the suit costs $300 or $10,000, if it doesn't fit, it will look horrible. That's why a good alterations tailor should become your best friend. Often, I hear complaints from clients about the cost of alterations compared to how much they paid for the suit. To this I usually reply, why did you spend a couple of hundreds of dollars on a new suit that makes you look and feel bad, when you can spend a little more to make it look amazing and make you feel powerful?

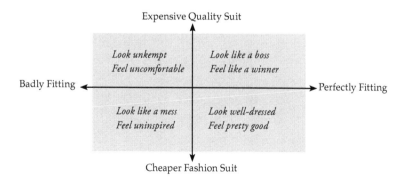

An experienced tailor will understand how a suit should fit, and they will spend time getting to know your body shape to work out and how to alter and style the suit to make it look uniquely tailored to you. When you first meet your tailor, make sure you discuss with them your shape, your style and your fit preferences, to avoid any mistakes or damage of clothing along the alteration journey.

If you are in Brisbane, *The Fitting Room* is the place to go for all of your suit alterations and maintenance needs. If not, here are some tips on how to find a good tailor.

Do they have good/genuine client testimonial and reviews?

The first thing to look for is genuine client reviews. Find out what types of alterations they specialise in. What is their level of customer service and how do they handle difficult situations? How they treat their clients is a reflection on how they will look after your order. What is their turnaround time and are they flexible to the client's needs? There is no use going to a tailor that takes two weeks to turn-around a hem. What is their average cost and is it comparable to other tailors at the same level? Most importantly, what is the quality of their work? These are all important factors to consider when deciding who is going to look after your precious garment.

Are they specialised in your garment?

When you walk into the store, have a look at the amount of work that's on their racks or in the workroom. What are the different types of work hanging there, and are they similar to yours? For example, if you want your suits altered, you would want to go to a tailor who specialises in suits. If you want a wedding dress altered, you would find a tailor whose shop is full of wedding dresses needing alterations.

Do they have evidence of their work?

If you are not sure, ask them to show you some of the work they have done before. For example: ask them to show you a jacket sleeve that they have finished shortening. This is a common alterations job, but few people can do it well. It is a good indication of the calibre of work that can be performed by the tailors. Make sure you look inside the cuffs as well, to check that no visible stitching, wrinkling, or frayed edges are apparent.

Who are their clients?

Are the other customers in the store of a similar demographic as you? If their regular clients are seeking out cheap deals, and you want quality alterations, then you are probably in the wrong place. Do they have partnerships with other businesses? For example: *The Fitting Room* is the contracted tailor for Hugo Boss, Canali, Brooks Brothers and dozens more clothing businesses.

Have they worked with this brand?

Ask the tailors if they have work with your brand of clothing before. Many brands make their garments differently, and some have special features. Make sure the tailor has worked with a range of brands and designs previously, and that they are able to maintain the specialty of your garment.

For example: surgeon's cuffs are functional buttonholes on the cuffs of jacket sleeves. Many high-end brands make their suits with surgeon's cuffs, and the sleeves can only be shortened from the shoulder of the jacket. This is an extremely delicate alteration, which can only be performed by highly experienced tailors.

How long have they been in business?

The history of a company is also an important element when choosing a tailor. Some companies can claim they have been in business for decades, but some crucial things to consider are:

* Who is the current owner?
* How long have they had this business for?
* What is their experience?
* Do they actually work in the business?
* Are they passionate about what they do?
* Do they take pride in their work?

Major franchises can claim to be a big operation with a long history; however, the staff that work there may not have the necessary experience to complete complicated alteration fittings, nor have enough vested interest to provide quality service.

Are they giving you honest advice?

The last point is also one of the most important points to consider. Is the tailor giving you honest advice? Do they listen to your requirements, and then help you fit the garment to *your* individual shape and style? Or are they giving you the basic offer they give to *every customer*, even if it is not a necessary alteration?

For example: a client brings in some trousers to Tailor One to have the legs taken in to be skin tight so that he looks more fashionable. The tailor listens and does exactly what the client says; however, the client ends up ripping the trousers on the first wear. Whereas Tailor Two will look at the body shape of the client and advise that the legs should only be slightly tapered because the trousers are not a stretchy fabric. By tapering the correct amount, the balance of the outfit is maintained and the client looks better as a result.

⌘

WHAT TO TELL YOUR TAILOR
BEFORE THE FITTING

You have a suit and you've chosen your tailor – so now it's time to get it altered. This is the most crucial step and cannot be skipped. Suits are generally not meant to be worn off the rack, as they need to be tailored for each individual's shape and size. Length, shape, waist, and width can all be adjusted. The key is to find someone who is experienced and understands suits to help you perfect it. This is not the time to be cheap, and to take it to your grandmother or auntie to get it hemmed up.

I often see junior office workers wearing suits as if they are a costume or uniform. They buy the cheapest suit possible that is in completely the wrong size, with the sleeves and trousers too long or too short. These people often stick out like a sore thumb and give the impression that it's their first day on the job, or that they're just there as an intern, or worse, dressed up in someone else's clothing.

Here are the important steps to having your suit professionally tailored.

Budget

Firstly, know your budget. Unless you are one of the few lucky 'standard-sized' men that can wear clothes off the rack, chances are you will need a few alterations. Are your limbs especially short or long? Is your torso narrower compared to your shoulders? Do you have very slim legs? If you know that you need some adjustments made to every suit, and how many changes you may need, then make sure you put away $100–200 for alterations. This is not something you can save on. There is no point in buying new clothes and wearing them if they are ill fitting. Everything looks better when fitted properly and complementing your shape.

Personal style

You should now recognise your personal style and know what makes you feel more like yourself when wearing a particular style. If you prefer to be comfortable and have a 'comfortable look', make sure the tailor does not taper the suit too much, and ask for them to ensure that there is enough room for you to comfortably sit down. If you want to look fashionable, then you may like your suit to be tailored to be a bit slimmer, which may in turn restrict your movement and be less comfortable to wear.

Make sure you communicate your preferences clearly to your tailor too. One of our clients brought in a pair of wide-leg trousers to be tapered in. He did not communicate to our stylist that he wanted a slim look. So we altered them to a standard straight-leg fit, and of course he was upset, so the alterations had to start again from scratch. It is also important to keep in mind that a suit is not a tracksuit. When you lift your arms or lean forward at a desk, make sure to unbutton your jacket. It will still be slightly restrictive, and you will not be able to do lunges or cartwheels, but such is the nature of a suit.

Occasion

Also, know where you are likely to be wearing the suit. Is it a professional setting or are you in a creative and more fashion-forward setting. Knowing why you need the particular suit will ensure that it is tailored appropriately for you and for the occasion. A slim-fit suit looks great if you work in fashion or creative industry. But if you work at a desk all day, it will not be comfortable and will not last long.

Timeline

If you need some major alterations to your suit, such as changing the shoulder width of the suit, or removing the pleats on trousers, expect it to take one to two weeks to complete. So make sure you allow the time for it, instead of running to the tailors the day before you need to wear the suit to a big meeting. Minor alterations, such as shortening trousers and shortening sleeves, will generally take around three to five days.

Expectations

Even though there are some talented alterations tailors out there, know that there is a limitation to what can be achieved via alterations. Once a suit is cut and made in a factory, simple alterations such as changing the length and tapering the seams can be an easy job. However, things such as changing the shape of the shoulders, reducing the size by more than two sizes, or increasing the size may not be achievable every time.

Some examples are if the jacket is too small in the shoulders, it can never be made bigger. If the jacket is too short, it cannot be made longer. If the jacket is more than 3 centimetres too small around the tummy, it can't be made big enough. It works the same with trousers – if they are too tight around the thighs and your behind, there is only a very minimal amount that can be let out.

If you wish to change the style of the suit, such as the shape of the lapel, adjusting the shoulder position etc., it will be considered a major alteration and the tailor should caution you about these types of alterations. Some tailors will try and say they can do it; however, without the experience, the suit may be damaged or the original shape completely lost. Make sure you get the right advice before going ahead with any reshaping.

⌘

ALTERATIONS: STEP-BY-STEP

A well-fitted suit is the ultimate expression of style. That's why having a tailor you can trust is essential to building a wardrobe full of incredibly comfortable suits that allow you to exude confidence. Here I will go through the step-by-step process of having a suit professionally tailored from beginning to finish.

Assessment = 5–10 minutes

The client is met with a stylist who has generally trained for 6–12 months full-time, before being qualified to fit a client's suit independently.

The stylist first asks the client what purpose this garment is for, whether it is for work (where it needs to be professional and comfortable), or if it is for fashion (where the suit is generally made tighter and shorter to show off the wearer's style). The stylist will look at the garment on the client and assess the overall fit, identifying areas that require improvement, such as length, size, fit and shape. The stylist is also able to provide advice on which is the best fit for each client, to complement the shape of the wearer and to meet the client's needs.

At this assessment, the stylist will determine if the size of the garment needs to be reduced, or if it needs to be reshaped in certain areas to sit better on the client's body. The majority of the time, it is possible to reduce up to two sizes on garments without altering the original style. Increases in size are often possible too, if there is enough seam allowance from the original make.

Fitting = 10–20 minutes

The stylist and/or tailor will then look at the construction and fabric of the suit and list the steps and work needed to perform the necessary alterations. By paying special attention to the client's shape, the garment is fitted on the client with pearl-head pins, each pin indicating where the finished seam will be, as well as the beginning and finish points of each seam adjustment.

Clients are encouraged to examine the fitting in the mirror, and pins are adjusted until the client is happy with the final fit of the garment. Make sure you tell your tailor if you feel the garment is too tight or not tight enough. Once the amount of work required to achieve the client's request is finalised, a cost for the alterations is provided and a time for collection or a second fitting is arranged.

Alterations = 3–7 days

Knowing how to use a sewing machine is not a rare skill; however, understanding the shapes and natural lines of garments and how they fit on the body is a talent that is refined through years of experience.

The tailor will first unpick the necessary seams and chalk out outlines where the new seams will be located. The pins in the garment indicate the desired size after alterations, and quite often it is not the exact amount to be altered along the seams. When chalking out new seams, the tailor takes into account the fabric integrity, seam allowances and adjustments for angle. For example: when 2 centimetres is required to be narrowed along the upper thigh, the sewing amount is adjusted to 1.25 centimetres to allow for the angled crutch seam.

At the same time, the tailor keeps in mind the overall shape of the garment and preserves the original shape and style as much as possible.

Other details to consider while sewing include: not distorting the stripes or check patterns on a suit; the tension of the stitching so as not to create wrinkles along the seams; the shape of the garment to be rounded to avoid sharp lines, and matching the thread colour to be as close as possible to the original. Every step is performed with the goal to have the finished garment looking as if it had never been altered.

Quality check = around 20 mins

A dedicated stylist (usually the same one that did the initial fitting) will check each finished garment for three things. Firstly, they will check that the alterations required are performed correctly and to the accurate measurements. Secondly, that the quality of the alterations meets the high standards expected, with the modified areas not being noticeably different from the factory standard. Lastly, that the whole garment is well presented, pressed, free of cotton and fluff, hanging on a suitable hanger, and all seams are closed. This is also a good time to pick up any new areas that might require fixing.

Second fitting = 10–15 minutes

From time to time, if the size of a garment is altered, another area that needs modification may become evident. Therefore, a second fitting may be required before the final alterations and the suit is collected. For example: at *The Fitting Room*, when we alter the size of the waistband on trousers, the length of the trousers may sometimes go up or down, requiring further alterations. Mind you, this basic change is usually picked up at the initial fitting by experienced stylists and accounted for.

For garments that require a major reconstruction, such as resizing blazers that are more than one size too big or too small, having a

THE SUIT BOOK

second fitting before finishing the jacket will help sort out any other adjustments that are required before finishing up the order.

Collection = 5–10 minutes

At the collection date, the client will be asked to try on the full tailored outfit. The tailor should look at the areas that have been altered to make sure each seam is sitting as it is supposed to. They will also look at the overall balance of the garment to check the whole outfit is sitting correctly on the body, and – most importantly – that it complements the wearer's shape. Clients understand that a perfectly fitting suit should make them look and feel incredible and that it ultimately increases the value of their suit.

So an investment of around 30 minutes, or two lunchbreaks, will make sure your suit is perfectly altered and styled to suit you. No more wearing ill-fitting suits that make you look and feel uncomfortable throughout the day. No more worrying about not being able to find a well fitting suit straight off the rack.

The Fitting Room regularly hosts pop-up tailors in major office buildings in and around Brisbane. You can contact us to find out if we come to your building. And if you're not in Brisbane, look out for other companies that offer this service in your local area.

⌘

99

HOW THE JACKET SHOULD FIT

There are two reasons why the fit of a jacket is so important. Firstly, it is the hero of every suit, so you want to get it right. Secondly, there's nothing worse than feeling uncomfortable in an ill-fitting jacket. With men having such varied upper body shapes, it is rare to find a jacket that fits perfectly. Sagging, bunching and rippling of the fabric are all signs that the garment needs some altering. The good news is that alterations are simple to make, but do try to avoid jackets that are too short in length, too small in the torso or too narrow around the shoulders, as letting them out is far more complex than taking them in, and not always possible.

Chest

The chest area is the aspect of the suit that people will generally notice initially, so it's important to get it right. When the lapel is popped open on the jacket, or pulling towards

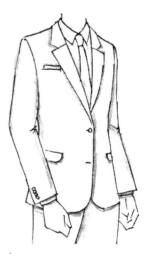

▶ A well fitting jacket

100

the sides, it means the jacket is too small. So I suggest that you go one size up and have the other areas adjusted to fit.

Waist

Structurally, the jacket's torso is one of the most complex parts of a suit. That means that if this part of the jacket doesn't fit snugly, there are plenty of ways it can be altered. When a jacket is too big and doesn't sit neatly against your body, it can be tapered through the back and side seams.

Turn to your side and look in the mirror. Check to see if the back panels are tapered to the shape of your body. The trend now is to have very slim-fitting suits, but it should not be so tight that it is pulling at the seams and making the vents flare open.

The perfect fit should be smooth and curved against the back, and the front panels of the jacket should hang flat when the buttons are done up. Tailors can taper the jacket torso to achieve the modern, well-tailored look. If you have a very lean torso, the darts in the front of the jacket can also be tapered in slightly for a fully customised look.

Some guys want to show off the hard work they've put in at the gym, and so they want the jacket to be fully tapered to hug their body. However, this can make them look top heavy, too curvy and lose all balance of a well-fitting suit. The suit should be structured, draping off the body, filling out hollows and hanging off protrusions, and balancing out the whole body.

Shoulder

Jacket shoulders are important to get right, as they do have a significant impact on the overall style of a suit. In the nineties, for example, wide shoulders were wildly popular, but now slim-fitting suits are back and this fit is far more flattering. If you happen to have a suit that is older but still in good condition, altering the shoulders is a simple way to modernise it.

In terms of fit, the shoulder seam should rest where your arm meets your shoulder. If the shoulder pads hang past your shoulder line or if dimples form at the top of the sleeve, this part of the jacket is too wide and needs to be taken in. When ripples form in the fabric around the shoulder seam at the top of the arm, the shoulders are too narrow and the fabric is being stretched as a result – you will also feel the restraint across your back, and this stretch will be noticeable. There is no option to make the shoulders wider.

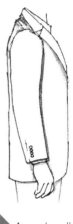

▶ A neck roll

The shoulders are the most delicate and expensive alteration done on a suit, therefore it is advisable to buy a jacket that fits very well across the shoulders. Should you need alterations, it is best left to the professional tailors like *The Fitting Room*.

Neck

Have you heard of your tailor talking about the squareness of the neck? All jackets come with wadding and shoulder pads around the shoulders. The pattern is usually tailored for 'average-shaped' shoulders. For sloped shoulders, a tailor can add padding to give you a more structured look. Some guys have very square shoulders (that's when your shoulders are almost at a right angle to your neck). In this case, you will find that most off-the-rack suits bubble at the back of your neck. This bubble can also be easily rectified by a few alterations.

Sleeves

Having the correct sleeve length shows that you pay attention to your attire and this is one of the easiest adjustments to make. If your jacket sleeves are too short, the jacket will look as though you've outgrown it. If they are too long, the cuff of your shirt won't be visible and your suit will look unpolished. The length and width of the sleeves can make or break an outfit. The cuff should sit just above the wrist bone, with 1–2 centimetres of your shirt cuff showing past the sleeve of your jacket. The width of the jacket cuff should comfortably wrap around your shirt cuffs, but it should not have enough room to fit in another hand. If you find your French-cuffed shirt is distorting the shape of your jacket sleeves, then your jacket sleeves are too narrow, and you may need to switch to a plain-cuffed shirt.

Length

The jacket should sit aligned to the end of your fly. However, if you wear your trousers lower or higher than normal, another indication as to whether the length is correct would be that the jacket lines up

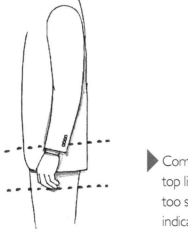

▶ Correct jacket length. The top line indicates the jacket is too short and the bottom line indicates the jacket is too long.

to the knuckles of your hands when they're relaxed by your sides. If the length is too short, it throws off the balance of the suit and makes the whole thing look too small and casual. If the length is too long, the wearer will look 10kg heavier and 5 centimetres shorter.

Golden rule

Always have your top jacket button done up when standing and undone while sitting. Buttoning your jacket while standing creates a cleaner silhouette, while unbuttoning it when you sit is more comfortable and prevents wrinkles forming. When standing, the bottom button on a two-button jacket should never be fastened.

Remove the extra bits

Make sure you remove all the white stitching on a suit jacket, i.e. on the shoulders, on the pockets, and usually there is stitching holding the vents closed. This stitching is there as an ode to traditional bespoke tailoring, where suits were 'basted' with white cotton threads by hand. Nowadays they're purely a decoration on brand-new suits, but need to be removed before wearing.

Often, I see guys wearing their suits with the vent stitch still attached. This is easy to miss, but it makes you look amateurish. Ensure it's unstitched so the vent is allowed to open and close with your movement.

Also remove the brand label on the outside of the sleeve. This is not a feature to be kept to show people where you bought the suit.

Front pockets and breast pockets can also be easily opened. Be careful not to use sharp scissors and damage the fabric, which will be expensive to mend.

Pick-stitch

You will often notice the visible stitching around the edge of the lapel, cuffs of the sleeves, and sometimes the hem of the jacket.

This is called pick-stitching. Traditionally, pick-stitch is done by hand, and it symbolises that the suit is handmade and shows off its prestige and the prestige of the man wearing it. However, now it is common practice on many off-the-rack brands, as automated pick-stitching machines became available. I still like the look of the pick-stitch, because it adds a bit of texture to the edging, and it holds the edges to be more flat.

Jacket fits

There are different types of jacket fits available from the stores when you are purchasing a suit. Knowing which fit is the best for your shape will save hours of trying things on that don't work, or spending lots of money on alterations for a suit that should have been a different fit to start with.

Classic fit

The fit of the jacket is made so the body of the suit is proportional to the shoulders. This fit flatters men who have squarish body shapes, where they have a wide waist and flat chest. These suits have wide front panels, which do not taper greatly towards the waist. This fit is also perfect for guys who have a wide chest, and the back panels can be slightly tapered to fit around the waist.

Slim fit

Perfect for guys who are very trim around the tummy but have wider shoulders. The waist area of these suits is extremely tapered and curved – able to fit guys with a inverted triangle body shape.

Wide fit

This is perfect for men with a bigger tummy. The front panels of these suits are wider, to accommodate for the extra girth. This means that men can button up their suit jackets comfortably, while the back panels still fit flat. This fit is perfect for round and triangle body shapes.

Long fit
Some brands make longer fitting suits for tall and slim guys who need a longer sleeve length or trouser length. A normal suit jacket sleeve can only be lengthened by 3cm, and trousers by 5cm. Therefore, having these longer cuts allow even the tallest of guys to buy a suit off the rack.

Short fit
Sleeves and trousers can be shortened; however, on a regular cut, if a tailor cuts off more than 10cm, the width of the barrel becomes too wide. The vents on the sleeve cuffs are also often lost. Having a short cut means that the suit features remain and are more proportional even after some shortening.

Jacket sleeve styles
There are a number of ways the sleeves of the jacket is finished. Each one slightly different, but can affect the cost of having it shortened or lengthened.

Plain sleeves with lining
This is when the fabric is smooth all around the cuff, with no visible split, or vent in the fabric. Plain sleeves are found mostly on female jackets, tuxedos, and on some overcoats. This is the most straightforward type of cuff to shorten, and the least expensive.

Standard sleeve with vent and buttons
When you buy a new suit, 80 per cent of the time it will come with 'shams', or decorative buttonholes on the sleeve cuffs as well as a fake vent. This particular stitching is found next to the button on the cuff, to imitate the look of a buttonhole. With this style, a tailor can shorten or lengthen sleeves at the cuff, as this stitching and the buttons are easily removed and can be replaced.

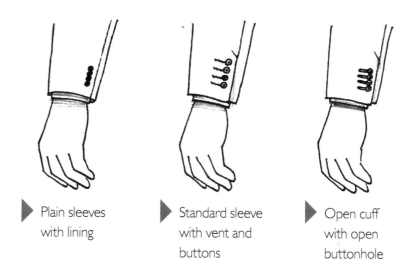

▶ Plain sleeves
with lining

▶ Standard sleeve
with vent and
buttons

▶ Open cuff
with open
buttonhole

Most of the time, the shams are not very noticeable (e.g. dark stitching on dark suits). In these instances, you can opt to not have the shams re-stitched after alterations, to save money. However, it is advisable to restore the cuff to its original look by having the buttonholes/shams stitched back on.

Open cuffs – open buttonhole
Open buttonholes are also called 'surgeon's cuffs'. Before the industrial revolution, all suits were custom-made for each person, and the sleeves were finished with functioning buttonholes and an open split. This was to ensure that the doctors could open the buttonholes to roll up their sleeves while performing surgery.

There are a few brands out there, such as Tom Ford, who only produce cuffs with fully functioning buttonholes. These may look more dressed up and make the suit look more expensive, but it also means it will cost more to have the sleeves altered.

From the cuff, tailors can only shorten or lengthen up to one centimetre, as the buttonholes cannot be moved. If more length is required to be taken off, a professional tailor can alter it f r om the shoulder of the jacket. It is a significantly more complex job, and only a few tailors would have the experience to perform it, so therefore it generally costs more than shortening from the cuff.

Open cuffs – buttonholes not cut open
This is the best option, where jackets come with the buttonholes stitched but not opened. The split is also sewn in a way to allow for conversion into an open button cuff. This style means you can try on the suit and only open the buttonholes if the length is perfect. Alternatively, you can have the sleeves shortened or lengthened from the cuff, and you can easily convert it to a surgeon's cuff later. Once the buttonholes are cut open, alterations of length must be performed from the shoulder.

Cuff buttons

Buttons can be sewn on the cuffs using three different styles – spaced, kissing, and stacked. Mostly, it is personal preference as to which style you choose, but kissing or stacked are the most common configurations.

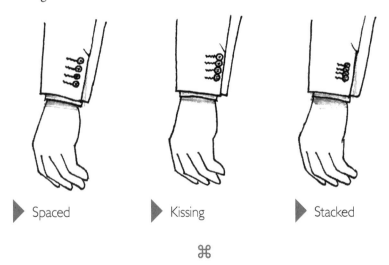

▶ Spaced   ▶ Kissing   ▶ Stacked

⌘

HOW THE PANTS SHOULD FIT

A good pair of trousers is a staple item in any wardrobe and the right fit will flatter your natural body shape. Investing a bit of time and money for alterations on your new trousers will elevate your look instantly.

Taper legs

A tapered leg suits most men, as it elongates the body and has a slimming effect, which is an important consideration if you are short and want to look taller. Like the length of your trousers, the width you choose will depend upon whether you prefer the classic wide-leg look or a modern tapered style. Often men are reluctant to try tapering, fearing it will end up being too tight and look unprofessional.

For a classic, professional look, taper the trousers from the knee down. The amount of tapering should be in proportion with your body shape, so that your pants are as flattering as possible.

Fashion-forward men like to taper the trousers to be figure hugging from the thighs all the way down to the hem. Although this look may look great when you are standing, it is often not practical for men who sit at a desk all day, and who need some room for movement. It is also

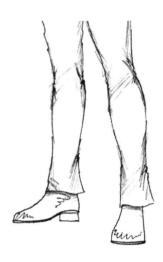

The trousers are tapered too much and the legs are too tight

not suitable for men who have muscular, short legs, no matter what fashion bloggers say.

The classic look of the pleat-front trousers is slowly coming back into fashion. The extra bit of fabric gives more room in the front of the trousers, which is perfect for guys with a larger behind and muscular thighs. Make sure the trousers are tapered towards the hem to still look modern.

Waist

To find the correct waist fit, there should be just enough room to fit two fingers in the back of the waist of the trousers. This allows for comfort when sitting down. If the waist is too big, fabric will bunch up under the belt and in the back of the seat, which looks extremely untidy.

The waist can be easily taken in or let out by up to five centimetres. Low-waist trousers may be fashionable, but a higher waistband elongates the leg and is more comfortable to wear – it also makes the wearer look taller. The waistband should sit on the natural waist just under the belly button, not under the tummy or on the hips.

Seat

The seat is the most important thing to get right, so make sure you are buying the correct size trousers for your behind. Look for the seat and crotch fit, which is the seam in the centre back starting from below the waistband that then goes around the crotch and up the front to the zipper fly. The curve of the seat should fit around your buttocks comfortably.

When the seat is too narrow across the bum, the front pockets will flare open and wrinkles will appear horizontally under the buttocks. When the seat is too short, it will ride up the buttocks. If the seat is too loose, it will look like you are wearing a nappy. It is far more complex to alter the shape of the seat and crotch than the waist of trousers. Therefore it's essential to try and find the right shape that fits you when purchasing trousers.

We once had a new client come to us to have his seat mended as it had ripped down the centre. I noticed that he had actually sewn press-studs onto his front side pockets to keep his pockets closed. This meant that the pockets flared when he had the trousers on. This is a classic example of when trousers are too tight across the seat, causing the seam to rip and the pockets to flare open. He would benefit from buying the next size up and have the waist sized to fit.

Saddle

Slimmer trousers also mean more wear and tear in the seat. We see a lot of men who damage their trousers in the crutch area due to rubbing between between the thighs. Installing a triangular piece of polyester or silk fabric in the crutch – a saddle – helps to reduce the rubbing, protects the fabric in the crutch, and it will increase the overall life of the trousers.

Trousers length

Many trousers are sold unhemmed, with the intention that clients will take it to a tailor to get it finished. Never wear your trousers without a proper hem, as the edges will fray, not to mention people will notice and wonder why your pants are not finished. Trousers can be easily shortened by as much as you need, or lengthened by up to 5cm. The ideal length is a small half break.

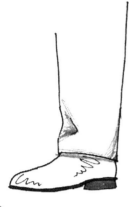

The Perfect Length

What most people don't realise is that there are a variety of lengths one can try. The key aspects are to make sure the length is matched to the width of the legs, the length should suit the wearer's body shape, and the look should be paired with the right outfit and for the right occasion.

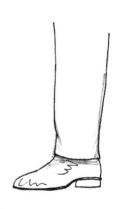

No Break

Cropped

This is a look not for the faint-hearted – you need to be fully committed to successfully carry this off. Keep the look simple with tailoring. Usually the trousers finish just above the anklebone and the hem does not touch the shoe at all. For this look to work, the trousers need to be very slim, especially towards the hem. This look can be worn with or without a cuff. The shorter length is not complementary to someone of a short stature. Instead, consider it if you are of a medium to tall height and of a slim physique. You can wear it with no socks and with quality loafers, or with dark block-coloured socks and dress shoes. No bright cartoon socks – please!

Half-break

The half-break is the look we recommend for most of our customers. It is perfect for slim or regular-fit trousers, as the hem sits over the rim of the dress shoes with one fold of the hem fabric at the front (the half-break). This look is modern yet safe, and it suits everyone, especially the vertically challenged men. This length covers the ankles completely, and it shows well-paired socks when the wearer sits down. There are some men who prefer not to have the break, but still want the trousers to cover their ankles. On these occasions, the tailor can slant the trousers to be slightly shorter at the front, thereby reducing the bubble (break).

Full-break

The full-break is the classic length for men favouring the more traditional look. It works well with straight or wide-leg trousers only. The back of the trousers comes right down to the end of the heel, and there are at least two breaks at the front. This look can be worn cuffed

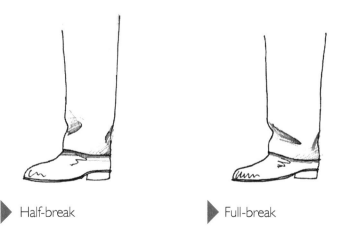

▶ Half-break   ▶ Full-break

or uncuffed. Hem tape can be useful to guard the fabric from being damaged due to the shoes rubbing against it. This look should be reserved for more formal occasions such as tuxedos and work suits.

When NOT to crop

There are a few instances that one should not wear the shorter trousers length. Cropped trousers are not for the vertically challenged, or those with muscular legs. The shorter length will make you appear shorter than you are. Instead, make sure the trousers have at least at a half-break, and that they are slightly tapered towards the hem.

Wrong cut

The most important aspect of cropped trousers is the cut. It must be fully tapered towards the bottom of the hem. If the trousers are a straight or wide cut, and flap around at the ankles, they will make the wearer appear as if they have outgrown their school trousers.

Types of hems

When clients come in to have their trousers shortened, the tailor will often ask them what kind of finish they would like on the trousers. I can hear you ask – 'Pants are pants, isn't there just one type of hem?' But actually, a simple pair of trousers can have numerous styles of finishing. Work trousers, jeans, tux trousers, gym pants – they can all be finished differently, using different sewing machines.

The following is a break down of the different types of hem finishes that are possible, and when each is appropriate.

Blind hem

The blind hem is the standard finish on most trousers. The hem is finished with an invisible stitch with a 5 centimetres allowance on the inside of the hem. A well-sewn pair of trousers should look perfectly smooth on the outside of the fabric, with no pulling or stitching showing through. Be careful not to put trousers straight in the washing machine, as the hem can unravel easily if not properly cared for.

Blind hem with half tape
A half tape is a piece of cotton ribbon that is wrapped around the inside edge of the hem on the back half of the trousers. This is used traditionally to protect the trousers' fabric from rubbing against your shoes. The cotton tape is only sewn on one of its sides and the ends are tucked into the side seams, giving it a very tidy and sophisticated look. The half tape is sometimes made in the same fabric as the trousers.

Blind hem with full tape
The most common tape is the polyester tape, and it goes all the way around the hem. Not only does the added material provide protection against the fabric rubbing against the shoe, it also helps provide extra weight, thereby giving the trousers a more structured look around the hem. Some brands have the tape fully hidden, sometimes 1–2 centimetres above the hem, while others place it at the edge. It is a signature look for Hugo Boss trousers to have the tape just peeking out from the hem of the trousers.

Cuffs
The cuffs on trousers add a degree of sophistication to an otherwise plain look. It is very common on old-fashioned suits, but it is coming back into fashion. Varying between 3.5 centimetres to 5 centimetres, the height of the cuff needs to be matched with different lengths of trousers. A small 3.5 centimetres cuff is suitable for a wide hem. Cuffs that have a width of 5 centimetres are perfect for slimmer and shorter lengths, but if the length is too long, there can be fabric bunching and look heavy on the ankles.

False hem
If you are a tall man, you will often hear tailors use the term, 'false

hem'. This is when a pair of trousers needs to be made longer by using the fabric allowance on the inside of the hem. We then add another piece of fabric on the inside to create a false hem allowance. This fabric is required so there is enough weight on the hem of the trousers to keep a nice shape. If you don't use a false hem, and have only a 1–2 centimetre hem, then the trousers may roll and not sit properly, thus looking very untidy.

Topstitch
The visible topstitch is used on jeans, casual pants and sometimes chinos. The fabric is cut and rolled twice, then sewn down with a plain straight sewer. The finish is one row of tidy visible stitching. Jeans typically have a 1 centimetre hem, and some chinos up to 4cm. The visible topstitching is stronger than a blind hem, and it will never unravel.

If you are ever unsure as to which hem you should have, just ask your professional tailor. It's better to ask them than risk damaging your precious garment. At *The Fitting Room*, we will always put back the finish that came from the factory, unless otherwise specified. And if we can provide a better outcome to make the garment look better, we will suggest an alternative.

⌘

HOW THE SHIRT SHOULD FIT

Imagine an important client or your boss walking into your office unannounced. You have taken off your jacket because it's too hot. You are in your business shirt with your sleeves rolled up because they are too long. The fabric on your collar is bubbly after being in the wash a couple of times, and the body of the shirt is much too large, ballooning around the sides with one side untucked. Is this the professional image you want to portray?

In Brisbane, it is too hot to wear a jacket all the time, so most men take it off during the day, exposing their ill-fitting shirts. Men often think that a shirt is not worth the effort to have altered, as it is worn under the jacket, and it is sometimes seen as a cheaper garment.

This is *not* the case!

A shirt should be one of the most important investments in your wardrobe. The fabric sits right against your skin all day, so it should look crisp yet feel soft. The fit should be tailored against your shape, the length correctly adjusted, and the hem should always be firmly tucked in, so you look well put together any time of the day.

There is a fine line between a well-fitted shirt and one that is too big. Unfortunately, many guys end up crossing that line because most of them struggle to find shirts off the rack that fit correctly. Most often, you might find that your sleeves are too long so they cover your hands, or that even the back of the shirt sits like a balloon and the armholes are halfway down your body.

It's essential that you ensure that all your shirts are just as well fitting as the rest of your outfit.

Here are three key areas that you must pay attention to, to look your best in your business shirts.

Sleeve length

In terms of length, the shirt cuff should just cover the wrist. Any longer or shorter and your shirt will appear ill fitting. While it's tempting to make your sleeves shorter to show off a nice watch, a far more sophisticated way to dress is to have a slightly looser shirt cuff that your watch will

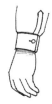

▶ Correct sleeve length

comfortably sit underneath. Once your shirtsleeves have been shortened, it's generally not possible to lengthen them again.

For a tailored fit, taper your sleeves gradually down the arm. Tapering sleeves to the correct width prevents bunching around the shoulder, elbow and cuff. To check the fit of your sleeves, pinch the fabric – it should be no more than 3 centimetres wider than the arm.

Single cuffs, French cuffs

There are single cuffs and French cuffs. Single cuffs are the basic dress-shirt cuffs, where the cuffs are one layer of stiffened fabric around the wrist. French cuffs are folded back onto themselves and secured with cufflinks. The French cuff looks more

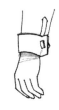

▶ French cuffs

sophisticated, especially when paired with well-chosen cufflinks. Keep your accessories classy and avoid cartoonish characters. Make sure the jacket sleeves are tailored to fit whichever shirt you are wearing.

Torso

Too many men wear their shirt more than one size too big. The first thing to look out for when selecting a size is the shoulder width. The seam where the sleeve joins onto the shirt should sit right on the edge of your shoulder.

Finding the right fit on the torso is a familiar struggle for many men, especially those who have wider shoulders and a slim body, as shirts that fit across the shoulders will come with a large fit on the torso. If that's you, make sure you select a *slim-fitting* shirt, and avoid shirts with pleats in the back. You should also have your shirts tapered down the side seams and have back darts created by your tailor.

For men with large midsections, a shirt with a box pleat at the back will give you the best fit. Men with slimmer figures should avoid box pleats, as the shirt will balloon too much around the waist.

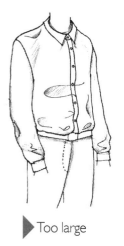
▶ Too large

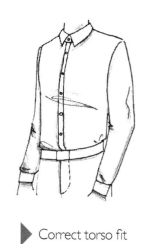
▶ Correct torso fit

Three centimetres of fabric on each side of the body is the ideal fit, though shirts can be tapered more depending on the look you are going for. Any excess fabric around the torso can be taken in using the side seams. If you notice buttons gaping at the front of the shirt, and the shirt is pulled taut against your skin, it is too tight.

Length

Most business shirts come in a longer length with a curved hem, because it is meant to be tucked in. Leaving it out makes the wearer look extremely untidy. For shirts that are to be worn out, make sure the hem is shortened and slightly straightened, so the hem sits just below the belt line.

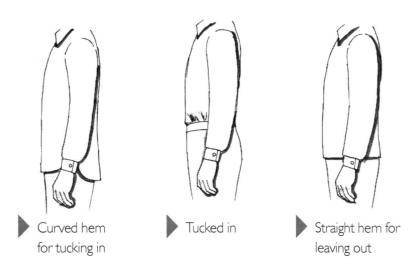

▶ Curved hem for tucking in

▶ Tucked in

▶ Straight hem for leaving out

Investing in a good shirt means you will spend less time ironing, and the shirt will last longer. When you are buying a shirt, the sizing range indicated doesn't give you much of a clue as to how it will fit. Usually the size just tells you the neck circumference and sometimes the sleeve length. Make sure you try each shirt on and find the brand and cut that makes the proportion that is most suitable for your shape, and then have the shirt tailored to fit you even better. Look for a quality high-weave cotton fabric, which is cool in summer and warm in winter.

⌘

MORE THINGS YOUR TAILOR CAN DO FOR YOUR SUIT

Trousers

- Put a silky saddle in your trousers to make them last longer.
- Mend ripped seams in trousers.
- Replace the fabric in the crutch of trousers if badly damaged over time.
- Replace or repair damaged pocket lining.
- Mend rips in jeans.
- Create rips in jeans.
- Create a frayed look on the hem of jeans.
- Turn jeans into shorts.
- Change the front of jeans from button fly to a zip opening.
- Make high-waist jeans into low-waist jeans.
- Change flares into skinny leg.
- Add or remove buttons for braces.
- Add or remove adjuster tabs.
- Make new belt loops if damaged.
- Add or remove cuffs on the hem.
- Replace a broken zipper.
- Add or remove the lining in trousers.

Shirt

- Change shirt from long sleeve to short sleeve.
- Remove pleats in the back of shirts to change into a slim-fitting shirt.
- Add a feature colour panel inside the collar of the shirt.
- Turn the collar inside out to hide damaged fabric.
- Add or remove pockets.
- Remove collar for a 'mandarin look'.
- Add button/buttonholes on collar peaks to hold them down.
- Change buttons to add a pop of colour to the shirt.
- Create new buttonholes to turn into a stud shirt.
- Make a panel of fabric to hide buttons on the front of the shirt to change the style.
- Slice in feature panels with different fabric on the body of the shirt to create a completely different look.
- Make new sleeve cuffs with feature colours to reflect your personality.
- Make French cuffs into single cuffs.
- Reduce the length of cuffs.
- Shorten the length of the shirt so it doesn't need to be tucked in.

Jacket

- Swap out the buttons to make it look like a sports coat.
- Add or remove shoulder pads to change the look of the jacket.
- Remove the half-lining to turn it into a lighter summer jacket.
- Change the lining if it's damaged.
- Add trimming around cuffs and lapels to turn it into a tux.
- Add decorative stitching around the lapels and edging of jacket.
- Change up the buttonhole colours on the cuffs of sleeves to make them into feature buttonholes.
- Add fabric or leather elbow patches.

- Open buttonholes on the lapel for lapel pins.
- Shorten the length of the jacket for a more youthful look.
- Make vent straps so that the vents don't flare at the back of the jacket.

Waistcoat

- Change the lining colour for a feature look.
- Change the shape of the neckline from straight to round.
- Change the length of the waistcoat.
- Change the buttons of the waistcoat to change the look.
- Add or remove waist adjusters in the back.
- Change the shape of the hemline to straight or angled.

Accessories

- Custom make bow ties and neckties with special fabric.
- Make pocket squares with special fabric.
- Sew down fake pocket squares in jacket pockets.
- Widen or narrow neckties according to the trend.

⌘

SECTION FOUR

HOW TO CARE FOR YOUR SUITS SO THEY LAST LONGER

'You can have anything you want in your life if you dress for it.'
Edith Head

HOW TO CARE FOR
A SUIT EVERY DAY

People often ask me why their suits get worn out after only a couple of months of wear, questioning that the suits are just not made like they used to be made. I believe the answer often just comes down to simple maintenance. Your suit is very hard working. After a long day at work, it has probably absorbed dust, sweat, heat, food and even skin. Therefore your suit deserves a bit of 'TLC'.

Here are some tips and tricks that I have collected over the years to help you maximise the life of your suit.

Airing it out

At the end of each day, hang your suit on a butler stand or an appropriately shaped coathanger. Keep your suit hung out in a well-ventilated part of the house overnight, such as the hallway or near a window, but out of sunlight. Give the suit time to dry out and the natural fibres will get a chance to go back into shape, looking good as new. Rotate your suits so you are not wearing the same suit two days in a row, and make sure you don't wear one more than twice a week.

Dry-clean

Remember, your wool suits should only be dry-cleaned by a professional. It's incredible how often we see clients bring in their ragged, shrunken trousers after they have thrown them into the wash, asking if we can fix them. Dry-cleaning usually requires harsh chemicals, which can dry out the natural fibres over time, so it is advisable to have a suit only dry-cleaned every three to six months, depending on how often you wear it. Any food stains should be acted on immediately by dabbing the stained area with a damp cloth. If you want the suit refreshed to wear to a big meeting or event, simply bring it in to *The Fitting Room*, or your local tailor, for a steam press.

Get two pairs of pants

If you are someone who needs to wear a suit every day, chances are you wear your trousers several days in a row. This means that the trousers always get worn out much faster than the jacket. Then you are left with a suit jacket, and good luck trying to find matching pants again in the shops after a couple of seasons. The simplest solution is to buy *two* pairs of pants when you are purchasing the suit. Most suit retailers should be able to offer this service, especially if you ask nicely.

Put in a saddle

As discussed previously, a saddle is a triangular piece of fabric, which is usually made from cotton, silk or polyester, that sits in the crotch section of the trousers. The saddle helps to reduce rubbing between the legs and the fabric, and it can also help to absorb moisture, heat. It is a common problem for trousers to be worn out in the crotch. In Brisbane, men prefer to buy suits in a thinner fabric to cope with the hot weather so the crutch wears out faster. While it is not a foolproof method, installing a silk/poly saddle will help the trousers wear down less quickly in the crotch area.

Get the right tools

Just like you brush your teeth at night, invest in a good soft bristle brush and give your jacket and pants a good brush down every night. This will remove lint, dust, hair, food crumbs and anything else that may have fallen on it during the day. Coupled with a good airing each night, you may not need to dry-clean your suit for six months at a time.

Mend straight away

As soon as there is a popped seam, a small fray or a moth hole, get it mended straight away. While the holes are small, they can usually be mended almost invisibly, and re- enforcements can be put in to prevent them from getting worse. If you leave it too late, the holes will become too big, making the mending very visible, sometimes even not possible. Don't let a small silverfish ruin your thousand-dollar suit. So after each wear, check your suit over for small damages and take it to your local tailor immediately for repairs if needed.

Storage

Mold, mildew, silverfish, and moths – these are just some of the culprits that will silently destroy your suit if not properly stored. After airing out your suit, and checking that it is completely dry, store it in a breathable garment bag that is made of a non-woven or cotton fabric, *not* plastic. The coat should sit on a proper hanger so the shoulders do not change shape over time. Also, invest in some cedar wood balls for natural critter deterrence. If you already have a silverfish or moth problem, then go for the heavy weights such as mothballs made of naphthalene and camphor blocks.

Don't use the pockets

I know it sounds silly – why have pockets if you are not going to use them? Well, just remember that constantly taking things in and out of your pockets, as well as storing large, sharp-edged objects such as phones and keys, will dramatically decrease the life of your suit. The pockets will get worn out and the edges around the pockets will fray. Opt for slim-line accessories that fit nicely into your pocket, or invest in a good-quality man bag.

Get the right size

There is nothing more damaging to the suit than wearing a size too small. As soon as you lift your arm to wave at someone, bend down to pick up something from under your desk, or take a big step out of your car, something is likely to split. While the slim-fit suit might be popular right now, is it worth it to have to buy a new suit more regularly than normal? Our suggestion is that you shouldn't be a slave to fashion but dress for your own shape, as everyone is different. Choose a suit that fits you comfortably, and then have key areas tapered to complement your body – such as tapering the legs or tapering the sleeves.

Be gentle

You have invested hundreds if not thousands of dollars into your suit, so look after it. Take your jacket off when you need to do some lifting. Take care when getting in and out of cars. A good trick is to keep your legs together as much as possible when getting out of cars, and try to sit *into* a car, rather than step into it and risk ripping your crotch seam. Don't keep your hands in the pockets of your pants if possible, and make sure your belt is the right width so it doesn't damage the belt loops.

Useful tools to have:

* A good clothes brush to use every day.
* A good ironing board and iron, as a cheap iron that doesn't work properly just wastes your time and may damage clothing.

- A garment bag that is big enough and doesn't squash your suits. The bag should be breathable, so it should be made out of cotton or non-woven fabric. It must not be plastic, as this may suffocate the wool. The plastic also becomes the ideal environment for bacteria growth and can promote the growth of mildew.
- Good hangers are essential. Coats should be hung on hangers of the right size, with rounded shoulders. Hang your trousers on 'velvet-covered trouser hangers' to avoid the trousers creasing and falling off the hangers.

⌘

WHEN TO CLEAN A SUIT

Aside from the everyday maintenance tips mentioned previously, the way you *clean* your suit will affect its longevity. So let's look more closely at how you should clean your suit, to ensure it lasts.

Airing your suit on a butler and brushing it after each wear will help to remove the food and dust accumulated from wear. Thanks to the bristles of the brush, they will get in between the fibres of the suit to get any dirt or skin particles out.

However, in addition to this, it is advisable to dry-clean your suit as soon as there are obvious food stains. You can also invest in a good steamer, which can help the wool get back into shape, and help to deodorise and kill off bacteria between wears.

When you need to dry-clean your suit, here's a behind the scenes breakdown of the process that's involved when the suit is at the drycleaners.

What is dry-cleaning

Dry-cleaning involves large machines that look like washing machines, but the drycleaners use a chemical solvent (perchloroethylene) to wash the clothes. The solvent is used in the machine at a controlled temperature, and the clothes are tumbled around like a normal washing machine while the solvent dissolves the dirt and soil. The solvent is then completely extracted and recycled, and the clothes are then dried at a maximum of 60 degrees before the doors are opened. The chemical can be highly toxic if inhaled.

Good drycleaners will use new chemicals or completely clarify the solvent between each wash. Some inferior cleaners may reuse the chemicals for more than one batch. If the stains are not removed during the first clean, more solvent sprays can be used, but these are stronger and risk damaging delicate fabrics. This is why you should use a quality drycleaner service.

Why are suits 'dry-clean' only

Water can damage the fabric and cause the wool to shrink and the colours to fade, and sometimes it can change the shape. Dry-cleaning does not damage the fabric like water does, and it prolongs the life of the garment in the long run.

How often should I dry-clean

Dry-clean a suit every three to six months to make sure everything is removed. However, when sugary items, such as food and drink, have stained the garment, and they are not removed immediately, the stain will oxidise, change colour and become more difficult to remove in the future. The same thing can happen with perspiration on silk lining – it is best not to store your suit long term without cleaning it first, as the silk will turn yellow with time.

⌘

LONG-TERM SUIT STORAGE

Again, I cannot stress enough the importance of hanging your suit on proper hangers before long-term storage, or you will risk damaging the wool, shoulder pads and the whole shape of the suit. Hang the suit in a proper garment bag that is breathable, such as non-woven garment bags, or calico cotton bags.

Don't forget to have the garments dry-cleaned first before long-term storage. This will help deodorise, get rid of sweat and food to prevent oxidisation, and it will also get rid of any moths/silverfish that may be living in it.

If you need to pack up your belongings to go away and have to put the suit in a storage unit or a friend's garage/spare room for whatever reason, it's then best to keep the suit on a shaped coathanger. Otherwise you can loosely fold it and wrap it in tissue paper inside a plastic box with air vents/holes, or in a suitcase. Never put clothing in cardboard boxes, as this is the perfect breeding environment for silverfish and moths.

⌘

MOTH/SILVERFISH PREVENTION

Every week we have clients bringing in their beloved suits with small holes. These holes can ruin the look of a suit, and if not mended, that once small hole can become a larger rip.

The holes are often caused by silverfish or moths, who love to feast on your suit's delicious fibres. Silverfish are small, silvery bugs that live in the crevices of drawers and bathrooms. They usually like to eat paper, sugar, glue in books, and sometimes clothes. Moths lay their eggs in damp dark places such as your wardrobe. When the larvae hatch, they come out and enjoy a buffet thanks to your wool fabrics. Mending holes caused by these little critters can be very expensive.

Here are some ideas as to how you can prevent these pests from destroying your clothes.

* Clean food stains immediately with a washcloth or by dry-cleaning.
* Make sure the garment is completely dry before storing.
* Airing it out will reduce smells and the dampness from sweat.
* Remove any cardboard boxes and newspaper in your wardrobe – these attract silverfish.
* Vacuum carpet regularly to remove any silverfish or larvae that may have fallen onto the floor.

- Rotate the wear of your clothes regularly, and shake them often so critters cannot attach or live in them.
- Make sure your garments are cleaned and dry, and then store them in good-quality garment bags.
- Moths and silverfish hate the smell of mothballs and cedar wood. So leave these around your wardrobes and swap them for new ones every six months. Have your house pest controlled every 12 months.

⌘

WHAT TO DO
IF THERE IS A HOLE/RIP

Your favourite suit jacket has a small rip, or there is a tear on your trousers, or what about that pesky moth that has gotten into your wardrobe and chewed a small hole in your favourite suit? What do you do?

Besides it being extremely frustrating when this happens, it can easily ruin the look of your outfit. So when is it an easy mend? And when should you give up and donate the suit to the salvos?

Here are the most common repair jobs I see on a daily basis, and if they can be repaired.

Split seam

Sometimes the stitching along the seams has just come apart due to an unfortunately angled movement, or the pocket has caught on a door handle. If the fabric is not damaged, you just need a machine stitch to fix the hole and re-enforce it to stabilise the area. This is the easiest repair and once done it will look as if it's never been split.

Rip in fabric

Rips can occur near pockets, knees, jacket sleeves etc. If the fabric is damaged and frayed, it can be darned. Darning is where a piece of fabric is patched under the rip to stabilise the area, and then stitching is

137

done over the rip to make it strong. The result is visible, but very strong. Depending on where the rip is, you may choose to have it darned so the suit can be worn again. Rips in the crutch, along pockets, near seams and under cuffs should be mended, as they're not too visible. However, if you get rips in the front of your jacket, the elbow area, and the front of the knee, these can be very visible after darning. You may try another option, such as invisible mending (see below), or it might be time to say goodbye to the suit.

Moth hole

The annoying little moths and silverfish absolutely love natural fibre. In Queensland, you will often find small holes appearing on your favourite suit or jumper. Luckily, these holes can usually be mended invisibly, to save destroying a whole garment. Invisible mending is when each fibre gets woven back into the fabric, so the finish is completely invisible. However, it is very expensive and takes at least a week. For one to two moth holes, it is worth spending around $100 for invisible mending, compared to buying a new suit. Holes that are close to seams or in hidden areas of the body can be darned with a machine for a quick solution. Larger holes may cost hundreds to repair and need to be carefully considered.

Crutch is worn out

This is caused by your thighs rubbing while you're walking. This is usually not due to inferiority of the fabric or its make, but it's actually because of the nature of the fabric and everyone's individual body shapes. The finer the fabric, the more likely the fabric will wear out. That's why you will often hear retailers asking you to only wear fine wool suits no more than one to two times per week. Some guys have close-set legs, and they will find that their crutch wears out more quickly. A tailor can darn it by stitching a large triangular piece of fabric to the damaged fabric inside, and this may make the trousers last another six months. The result is visible, however, and the pants will feel stiffer, but the area will be stronger.

If the fabric is beyond damaged, then a tailor can cut out the fabric and replace it with a new piece. There will be a diamond-shaped seam in the crutch area, but this cannot be seen if you are standing or wearing the trousers. However, this fabric may still wear out over time if this is a common occurrence for your shape. Installing a satin saddle may slow down how fast the trousers wear out.

Hem fallen down

Trouser hems are usually hemmed with a machine that shows almost no stitching on the outside of the fabric. This is called an invisible hem. This type of hem comes apart very easily. This does not mean that the making of the trousers is inferior, but it could also be purely bad luck or being too rough with the trousers. With the right agitation, pulling or sometimes roughage, the seam can easily unravel and the hem can come down. It can be simply fixed by taking it to a tailor and having them run it in the hemming machine a few more times.

If you know your hems tend to fall down, pay a bit more and ask for the hem to be hand-stitched. This will still make the hem invisible and less likely to fall down. Keep in mind though that because it is hand-stitched, it will take more time to complete and will cost more. Hand-stitch is recommended on very fine fabrics that show stitching on the outside of the fabric if a machine is used.

Belt loops worn out

This is another very common occurrence on work trousers due to the belt rubbing on the fabric. The belt loops can be easily replaced by making new ones. If you have the cut off hem from when you first bought the trousers, a tailor can use that so the loops look exactly the same. Alternatively, the tailor can find a very similar colour to make new belt loops.

Pockets worn through

Guys tend to put a lot of things in their pockets – keys, coins, phone and wallet. Cotton pockets can often get worn through with overuse. The pockets can also be easily replaced or re-enforced by adding new cotton fabric.

Lining broken

The lining on trousers and jackets can get worn out over time, especially near the pockets, armholes and sleeves. Lining can be easily mended and is worth the effort if the suit is still in good condition, as it is inside the jacket and cannot be seen. If it is badly damaged, the lining can even be completely replaced to increase the longevity of the suit.

Zipper broken

Another common repair is fixing the zippers. Guys need to use their zippers many times each day, so it's no wonder it's one of the first parts of the trousers to get damaged. Zippers can be repaired or replaced for under $40, but please be careful with the fabric around it, for if you are too rough or in a hurry and rip the fabric, it will require darning, which is very visible.

When to chuck your suit away
* When the rip is somewhere very obvious and longer than 5cm.
* When the fabric has thinned so much due to wear that it is shiny and out of shape.
* When there are multiple moth holes and rips.
* When the fusing has come apart and the jacket has bubbled.

⌘

140

WHY THE CROTCH WEARS OUT AND HOW TO PREVENT IT

Many of our clients complain about the fast rate at which their trousers are damaged compared to ten years ago. They immediately assume that garments are just not made sturdy enough like the 'old days'.

So let's break down the reasons why your trousers keep wearing thin at the crotch, how to prevent it, and if all that fails, how it can be fixed. This is one of our most popular blogs and gets at least 5000 reads per month – that's why it gets its own chapter!

Reasons

Thighs

Muscular or large thighs, and a prominent behind, are the number one reasons for wearing out the crutch. This means the legs are usually touching when you walk, rubbing the fabric with each movement and thereby thinning it over time. This is not something you can change. Other reasons could be due to your gait, the shape of your legs, and how you walk. For example, someone with 'O-shaped' legs is less likely to rub their thighs as they walk, unlike someone that is slightly 'pigeon-toed' – their thighs will naturally rub together as they walk.

Trousers too tight
In the pursuit for high fashion, a lot of men are wearing trousers that hug their buttocks. This may look great in photos and when standing, but it is not comfortable when sitting. Prolonged sitting can actually strain the fabric around the crotch. Movement will then further damage the fabric, causing tears and holes to appear.

Fabric too thin
The finer fabrics, such as Super 160s, are beautiful to look at and feel wonderful to touch. However, this also means that the fabric will wear out faster.

Prevention
Saddle
This is a triangular layer of fabric, doubled layered and attached to the crotch of the trousers. Many high-end trousers may have a small cotton saddle sewn in the trousers to help absorb moisture through the day. We often install a large version, made of a poly/rayon fabric that is usually used as jacket lining. This extra layer has a number of benefits for the wearer – it reduces the friction from the legs rubbing against each other, absorbs moisture through the day and takes it away from the trousers' fabric, and it prevents the inseams of the trousers from rubbing against the legs.

By installing a saddle on every pair of new trousers, it helps to prolong the life of the trousers. This way is more economical than mending or replacing the trousers, especially when you have a matching suit jacket, and especially if the same trousers are no longer available for purchase.

Get the right size
One of the main things to look out for when purchasing new trousers is the crotch length. This is the seam that runs from the back of the

waistband down and around to the end of the zipper at the front. The crotch seam is one of the most important features of the trousers and comes in a variety of lengths and shapes. If the crotch seam is too short, or if the seat and thigh area is too tight, you are more likely to rip the inseams and create a big hole in the bottom.

Men with muscular behinds need to look for high-waisted trousers with a long crotch seam that curves nicely under the buttocks, without creating a 'wedgie' look. There must also be a generous amount of room in the thigh area to allow for movement. This is because there is often not much fabric in the seams around the thighs and seat area and therefore the area can't be made bigger. Go for the right size that will accommodate your seat and thighs, and ask your tailor to taper the waist and legs to fit. Men with smaller behinds can wear high or low-waisted pants and have the crotch seam shortened to complement the body.

Re-enforced crotch

If your seat is wearing out regularly, because of your shape or walking style, have your trousers re-enforced while they are still new. As previously mentioned, tailors can add a piece of fabric onto the crotch area to make it thicker and more hardy, as well as adding in a saddle.

Be careful

A lot of guys don't realise that tailored suits are not to be worn while exercising, cleaning under the desk or 'horsing around'. The fabric generally has no stretch, so if you decide to have a bit of fun on Friday afternoon, and try to leap frog over your mates, your trousers *will* rip.

Airing out

Moisture and bacteria from the body can make the fabric brittle over time and become damaged more easily. At the end of the wear, hang up your suit and trousers in a well-ventilated area so they have a chance to dry properly and go back to their original shape. And even consider investing in a retro-looking 'butler stand' and prepare your outfits the night before.

Dry-cleaning
Jackets should be dry-cleaned every three to six months (or immediately if stained), and trousers should be dry-cleaned every five to six wears or when they become smelly. Try and buy two pairs of trousers with each suit so you have a spare pair to rotate with.

Fix

Mend area
Many men don't realise that garments can be mended and darned when damaged. As you now know, if the fabric on the crotch area is simply thinned or beginning to fray, tailors can re-enforce it by adding a piece of fabric under the hole and stitching it down strongly. The result will be slightly visible under the behind, but not visible when you are standing.

Replace fabric
Sometimes clients bring in their trousers when the holes are more than 2 centimetres wide and the fabric is paper-thin – this is when it is too late for mending. We can, however, cut out the damaged area and replace the whole area with a new piece of fabric, and then install a saddle. The finish is very tidy and comfortable. The challenge though is in finding an identical piece of fabric that is large enough for the area. Therefore, it is a good idea to keep the cut off from your trouser hems when you have them altered at the purchase time.

I read an article in a prominent men's fashion magazine that I could not disagree with more. In the article, it advised men to throw away their jeans and trousers once a hole appeared in the crotch, because it would be too expensive to fix.

There are several things wrong with this suggestion.

Firstly, mending is not expensive compared to the overall expense of a quality pair of trousers – in fact, mending is a fraction of the price. To suggest that the mending is expensive would mean they are encouraging men to purchase trousers that cost less than an iPhone cover, or a bottle of wine. Cheaper, fast-fashion garments may look glamorous, but these particular outfits generally only last several wears before they are damaged or get dumped. They are also more often than not produced in an unethical and unsustainable fashion.

How many wears do you get out of each piece of new garment you purchase? When was the last time you had a garment mended instead of throwing it out?

We recommend that each person purchases high-quality ethical fashion, and by looking after it well, it *will* last the distance. It may cost more in the short term, but with a small investment in damage prevention, a well-made garment will pay itself off with the number of wears you get out of it.

⌘

SIX HABITS THAT ARE SECRETLY RUINING YOUR SUITS

You might find that you are guilty of one, or a few, of these 'habits' when wearing your suit – and that's understandable, as they are easy things that can go unnoticed *until* you witness them affecting the life of your precious suit. So make a note of the following, and if possible, be mindful and try to stop yourself from doing them in the best interest of your 'investment'.

Hanging on by your belt loops

Many men tend to hitch their trousers up by hooking their fingers in the belt loops. This places extra strain on those small loops, causing your belt loops to wear away and even tear the fabric of your trousers. Make sure your trousers are the correct size by having them professionally sized by a tailor, so you won't need to hitch your trousers up all the time. If you do need to adjust them, pull on your trousers by the sides of the waistband, as this area is wider and stronger, and has more support. If your belt loops are getting worn out, a tailor can mend or make new loops for your trousers.

Stashing your wallet and keys in your pants pocket

Here at *The Fitting Room*, we often mend the pocket opening on trousers every week due to bulky wallets and keys damaging the pocket. Overuse of these pockets not only wears away the lining of your pocket, it may also damage the trouser fabric around your hips, leading to regular mending and ultimately shortening the life of your trousers. Filling your pockets with weighty items can also make you appear bulky when walking, push out the seams of your jacket and ruin the sleek overall look. To minimise fabric damage, keep your essentials in your bag.

Not having a satin saddle in your trousers

This usually means your jacket will outlive your trousers. One of the most commonly damaged areas we do mend is in the crotch, caused by wear and tear to the inner seams from movement. The life of your trousers can be extended by installing a satin saddle to give your inner seams more strength for general movement and also to reduce friction. Tailors, like us at *The Fitting Room*, should have several satin saddle sizes ready to install on your trousers.

Not airing out your suit after wearing

Not airing out your suit after wearing it may trap moisture and odours into the fabric, which creates an environment well suited to the development of mould and mildew. Air your suit out overnight, before hanging it in a dry ventilated wardrobe. Additionally, cedar wood, mothballs and camphor can assist in keeping your fabrics safe from insects. Refresh your suit by dry-cleaning and deodorising it semi regularly.

Wearing your trousers too tight

Slim-fitting trousers are on trend right now, but when is it too tight? Besides making you feel restricted in movement, slim-fit trousers put more pressure on your trouser seams than usual, and making your pants more prone to ripping at the seams. The aim is to have enough movement in the seat and thigh area while bending and sitting, and have the legs tapered towards the hem. Trouser waist/seat/legs can generally be adjusted to suit your changing needs, and tailors can help you check your trouser fit to ensure they're the right size and look on point.

Not hanging your jacket up when not in use

Your jacket's most important feature is the structure and shape. By not hanging your jacket up on a coathanger, you risk irreversible damage by crushing and wrinkling the fabric layers, and having the shoulder pads and wadding go out of shape. Jackets should be kept on wide jacket hangers that can hold the weight and preserve the shoulder shape. Invest in premium hangers and you'll always look sharp when donning your jacket.

⌘

SECTION FIVE

DRESSING WELL

IS A MIND SET

'*Dressing well is a form of good manners.*'
Tom Ford

HOW TO BE A 'MODERN GENTLEMAN'

In the Oxford Dictionary, the traditional definition of 'gentleman' is: 'A chivalrous, courteous, or honourable man, the term denoted a man of a good family (especially one entitled to a coat of arms) but not of the nobility'. As well as, 'A gentleman of noble birth, high social status and does not have to work'.

The term 'modern gentleman' carries a different meaning nowadays, and it can be interpreted various ways. It no longer means that someone is of 'good birth', and that they don't work. Nor does it denote that the person is of a higher status than another.

In the modern day, it is more reminiscent of someone who carries good manners and earns respect from others via his actions.

The word 'manners' has changed meaning over the years. If you attempt to order food for a lady or pull out her chair, you may be seen as domineering and sexist, unlike the yesteryears.

Here at The Fitting Room, we believe in some basic rules for being a 'modern gentleman' – a gentleman should:

* be well dressed and well groomed;
* have high standards for themselves;
* not curse easily in normal conversation;

- have good manners and is considerate of others;
- be worldly and well-read;
- be open minded, yet not brag about their opinions or force it onto others;
- be true to their word;
- be non-judgmental, no matter their background and opinions;
- have self-respect and respect for others;
- admit when they are wrong and learn from their mistakes.

Being a gentleman should be something you aim to be throughout your own personal journey of growth. It is not a status, but rather a personality trait developed over time and comes with maturity. Being called a gentleman should not be because you are well bred, or because you fulfill one or two of the criteria by appearance. When you are referred to as a gentleman, it should come as an honour, as it is a reflection of who you are as a person.

⌘

HOW TO BEHAVE IN A SUIT

Now that you have the 'attire' part of being a gentleman down pat, it's time to make sure you are well rounded and educated in the other aspects of being a modern gentleman.

Etiquette/ modern manners

By practising the art of conversation, learning the ins and outs of modern manners and mastering contemporary etiquette, you will feel more confident talking to everyone from new colleagues to old friends. A gentleman should always make the other person feel comfortable and welcome in a conversation.

To polish off the 'ambience' of your suit, it's now time to think about learning some traditional manners, and how you can incorporate them into your modern-day life. Gone are the days of opening the doors for women, or trying to stand on the edge of the sidewalk when walking with women. It's still important to act with grace and consideration for others, but men and women should be treated equally.

Table manners are also very relevant – waiting for everyone's food to come before eating, never starting to eat before the host, understanding the uses of your utensils and wine glasses etc.

Phone manners should be carefully considered when in the company of others – keep it on silent (most of the time), don't browse the net/social media, check your messages discreetly if you have to, and excuse yourself if you need to take a phone call.

Learning how to act like a grown man includes introducing yourself confidently to others, introducing acquaintances to each other by describing them with a short sentence, having a firm hand shake, using an appropriate tone and volume of your voice in public, and not cursing in front of people you don't know well, especially in work situations.

You should also learn to compose yourself in public and be 'media ready' in any situation, such as emergency presentations to clients/team members, and being well dressed so you can attend or lead impromptu meetings.

Culture and general knowledge

From food to art to travel, culture seeps into every part of our lives. Some knowledge to acquire includes: how to choose whiskey and order wine, the differences between cuts of steak, knowing some current affairs, understanding the history of different countries and cultures, appreciating art, and dressing for different occasions. Covering these such aspects will not only boost your own confidence when socialising with others, but it gives others a understanding that you are cultured, well learned, open minded and able to hold conversations with different people.

Structure

Until you are in a position to hire your own personal assistant, you need to be on top of things. Learn how to organise your own finances and maintain a productive mindset. Manage your work-life balance effectively. Keep healthy by having a good diet, exercise regularly and be mindful in all situations.

By arming yourself with all the above knowledge, you will become a more well-rounded person. You will find that you will have more confidence in all of your pursuits and all kinds of doors will open for you.

⌘

THE RETURN ON INVESTMENT
WHEN YOU ARE WELL DRESSED

I can't stress enough the fact that having a power suit and dressing well will give you many years of good 'return on investment' (ROI). When you are well dressed, you are more likely to be trusted. You will appear to be successful, and because of that appearance you will set yourself in the right mindset, and become more successful. You will be taken seriously, and you will be admired and respected by others.

But that's not all, as there can be a diverse array of positive changes in your life if you take care in dressing well and appropriately. Here I'll share some of the changes I have seen occur to my clients over the years.

Ryan first came to *The Fitting Room on Edward* ten years ago. Having won a national prize in export planning, he was invited to an event with the Prime Minister of Australia, so a new suit was justified. After purchasing an off-the-rack Armani suit, his friend told him to go to *The Fitting Room* to have it tailored.

This was his first alterations experience, and he didn't know what to expect. He said, 'Mylene (the manager) fitted me in the suit, advised me on the alterations required to look good, and had the suit ready well before I had to fly to Melbourne. I had never had a suit that fitted so well, it looked like it was tailor-made for me.'

Having a lean build, it is often difficult to find slim-fit clothing. After finding *The Fitting Room*, it became a habit of his to have all new purchases adjusted. With each alteration, he was learning more about fashion, the fit, stitching and style.

'I now know about box pleats, darts, and the difference between a slim leg and baggy leg pant. I soon re-assessed my clothing, and it became a habit to ensure my outfits were styled to suit me. I found that understanding more about a good fit changed the way I handled new clothing, and I even started to re-think my older pieces in the wardrobe.'

This included a designer camel-hair trench coat that was handed down to him, but he had never been able to wear it. *The Fitting Room* completely changed the cut of the length, sleeves, and the style. The trench coat is now a beautiful feature piece in his wardrobe.

'I receive compliments every time I wear it out,' Ryan said. 'Having *The Fitting Room* on Edward on my side, I never have to miss out on purchasing something I love, just because of size or fit. When I get compliments on my clothes now, I know that "fit" is one of the main reasons. I have recommended *The Fitting Room*'s style and clothing alterations services to many of my colleagues and friends, and many of them are now also addicted to well fitted clothing.'

Another recent client is a very sharp dresser. He came to us to have a new sports jacket tapered to take on his European family holiday. When he came back, he showed me all the photos, where he was impeccably dressed in each one. The best story he told me was when they were visiting a busy square in Italy, and there was a couple getting married. One of the family members pulled my client aside in a panic and asked him if he could please help the groom with tying his tie.

My client not only helped the nervous groom sharpen up his look, he ended up fixing the 'look' of the whole wedding party and their guests. The couple was so grateful that they invited my client and his family to join their wedding celebrations. My client ended up making amazing new friends. This only happened because he was dressed in a sharp, casual suit, wearing chinos, boots, a fitted-shirt, a bright sports jacket and a well-paired pocket square (yes, even on a family holiday).

One of my best clients is the managing director of a high-end menswear retailer in Brisbane. He said, 'It doesn't matter if it is 36 degrees outside, I never go to work without a properly fitted jacket on. What you wear every day is your suit of armor. Putting on a properly fitted outfit every day translates into your work. If you are wearing thongs and shorts, you feel crap and sloppy. If you wear a sharp suit in the morning, it will translate into your work, improve your confidence and increase your productivity. I dress a lot of very successful men, and they all understand what a good suit does to their image. To dress for success, the price tag of the suit is not the most important detail. Make sure your suit is fitted properly, styled with the right accessories and suits your shape. There is nothing worse than an ill-fitting suit. It is uncomfortable, distracting and will decrease your overall performance. Also, I would never recommend something for a customer just to follow fashion. Clothes should fit each person's style and shape.'

There was a man who used to work at a major telecommunications company, in a middle management role, and who left for another job after a few years. He then went back to the same company 18 months later, applying for and being accepted back into a higher position, with $100,000 more in his salary. When asked if he had gained more qualifications, skills or experiences, he said, 'No, it was nothing like that'. He simply interviewed in a bespoke three-piece suit, which was perfectly tailored to his body. This suit gave him confidence, power, and the air of knowing something that no one else knew.

I also know a very prominent business coach and keynote speaker who invests the time and money to make sure all his clothes are perfectly fitted, perfectly styled, and that they reflect his personality and purpose. He says that once he puts his outfit on, he feels like he is stepping into a high-performance vehicle. He moves with conviction; he communicates with clarity; he performs better and faster, and he feels impactful. He swears by the fact that dressing well in an appropriate suit gives him the extra edge he needs to carry out his job more effectively and successfully than if he didn't put as much focus on his outfits. And when he dresses well, he feels confident, and therefore his clients feel his positive vibes and this is integral to his career.

Recently, I was lucky to attend the book tour of famous American author, David Sedaris, in Brisbane. We had a little chat after the event, and I told him about my job and this book I was writing. He became so excited and started to tell me his story. A few years earlier he had a bespoke jacket made by a top tailor at Savile Row, London. It was the first time he had had something made just for him, and he couldn't stop raving about how amazing that jacket looked on him, and how it made him feel. He was convinced that it made him become more powerful, successful and confident. And he acknowledged that it was completely different to wearing off-the-rack clothing and trying to fit into it. From then on, he became addicted to tailored clothing.

⌘

FINAL WORDS

I do hope that this book has helped you understand the power of your 'power suit'. And if I could add some final words, they would be:

* How you dress is directly correlated with how you feel, and your confidence level. We all have a couple of outfits that feel like a 'suit of armor', making us feel strong and confident. And we also have some that make us feel less confident about ourselves. So why isn't every piece of our wardrobe a confidence booster?
* Instead of wasting time feeling deflated in badly fitting clothing, use the tools and tricks in this book to dress for the best version of yourself.
* A tailored fit never goes out of style.
* You don't need to spend a fortune or waste too much time in order to look and feel good.
* Quality over quantity – take your time when building a good-looking and valuable wardrobe.
* There are ways to alleviate the pain of buying and altering a suit, by understanding your own body, style and what's on offer to purchase.

- Do what you can to avoid fashion and social faux pas.
- Dress for the job you want.

What's next

Having read this book, remember:

- Don't feel like you need to rush out and start shopping straight away.
- Go through your wardrobe and pull out what you've always felt uncomfortable in. Chances are it may just need to be altered and restyled. Minor repairs can also be done to give your 'old favs' a new lease on life.
- Bring any garments into *The Fitting Room* to be assessed, if you're not sure.
- You can arrange for a call out to your office and home, if you can't get to us (Brisbane CBD only).
- Go to our website and download *The Fit Guide* and join the mailing list for up-to-date content.

Further information

Get your suits fitted and maintained at
www.thefittingroomonedward.com

Learn how to be a modern gentleman at
www.themoderngentry.com.au

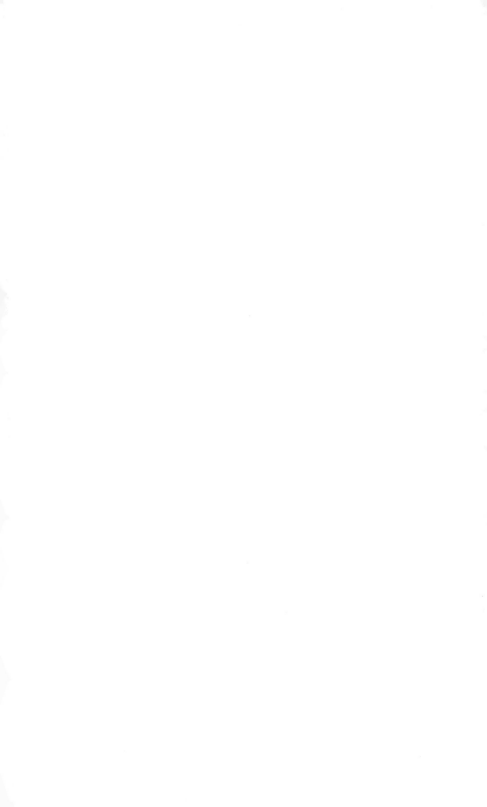

20066155R00102